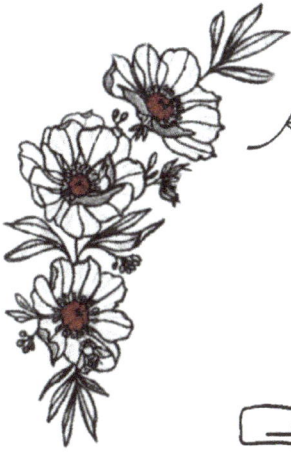

A Mountain In My Heart

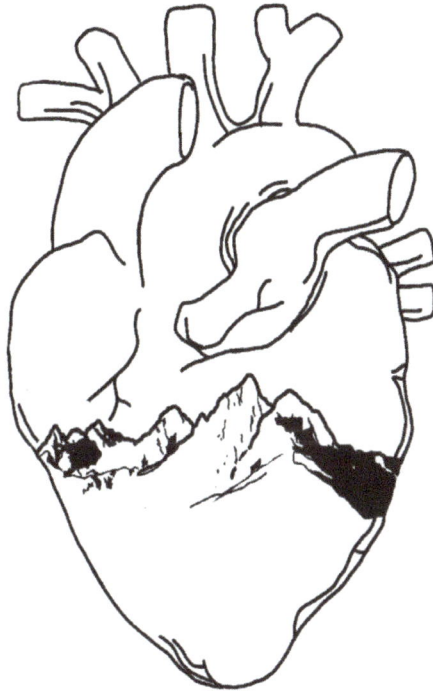

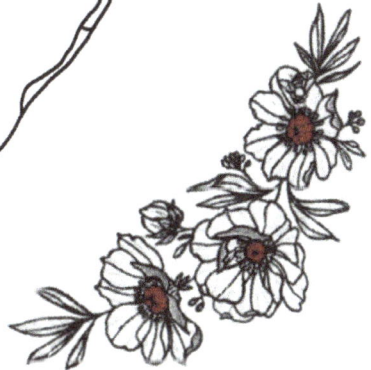

By Rosie Jarman

First published in the United Kingdom in 2023 by
The Choir Press

ISBN 978-1-78963-411-2

No matter how hard the past,
You can always begin again.
Buddha

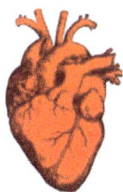

Contents

Dear Readers,

This book is here to help you to understand cancer and gives you tips and stories that I hope you find helpful. It also tells you about my journey and how it all started.

Quick Facts:

1 in 2 people will get Cancer in their lifetime – NHS UK (2022).

There are more than 200 types of cancer – NHS UK (2022).

In the UK there are around 3755 young people diagnosed with cancer each year. That's 1645 children (aged 0–14 years), 2110 in teenagers, and young adults (aged 15–24 years) – UK Health Security Agency statistics (15/03/2021).

There are almost 1.5 million people caring for someone with cancer in the UK – Macmillan.org (2016).

Across the age ranges, around 375,400 new cases of cancer are diagnosed in the UK each year (2016–2018). Around 167,142 people will die from the disease – Cancer Research UK (2022)

Early detection is key to saving lives, if something doesn't feel right get it checked.

"The only thing you can do is to fight
through your diagnosis …
And stay strong,"

Rosie Jarman 12/2021

Introduction

My name is Rosie Jarman, and before all this I was a perfectly healthy 14-year-old. I live in a small town in Wales with my mum, dad and sister. I was diagnosed with a rare heart cancer called High Grade Undifferentiated Pleomorphic Sarcoma (HGUPS) back in October 2021. I will explain more about it on page 62.

What brought me to the hospital originally was that I had COVID back in July, I was not keeping my food down and was not drinking as much. We thought I was dehydrated but then I was losing my breath when I was walking up the stairs and had started sleeping more upright. My mum took me to the GP surgery and after a couple of return visits they thought I had A-typical pneumonia because the GP heard crackling in my chest. They sent me to the hospital for an assessment which led to further assessments, resulting in a rush to London for emergency Open Heart Surgery. See page 6.

Hearing the words "you have cancer" filled my head with so many questions, like 'am I going to die?', 'what happens next?', 'what cancer do I have?'. They didn't know what cancer I had at that time because it was so rare.

I would never have actually thought that I had cancer and would lose my hair because of it. Now it is part of my story.

I have met so many amazing people on my journey and made so many new friends. Many have experienced similar treatments that I have/am going through although I have not met anybody who had to have open heart surgery to remove their cancer.

Having gone through that experience is hard, but you have to remember to try and stay positive even though at times you might not feel like it.

Before Diagnosis

My family and I would go out almost every week on walks and go camping when we could. I would also go out with my friends on shopping trips, walks etc.

Last year I did four Duke of Edinburgh expeditions up two mountains. I am also in the RAF cadets so did two expeditions with them and two with school not knowing at the time I was functioning on less than three-quarters of my heart.

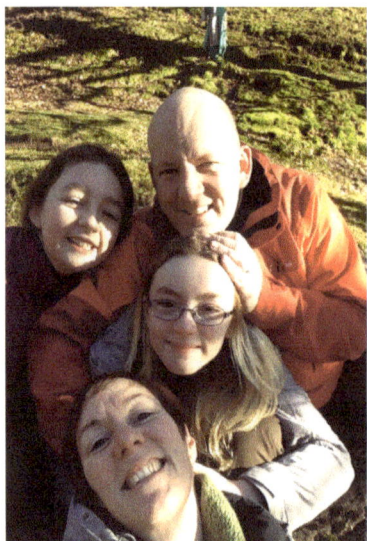 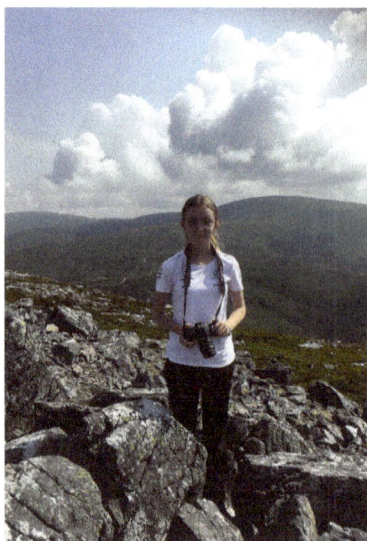

My family

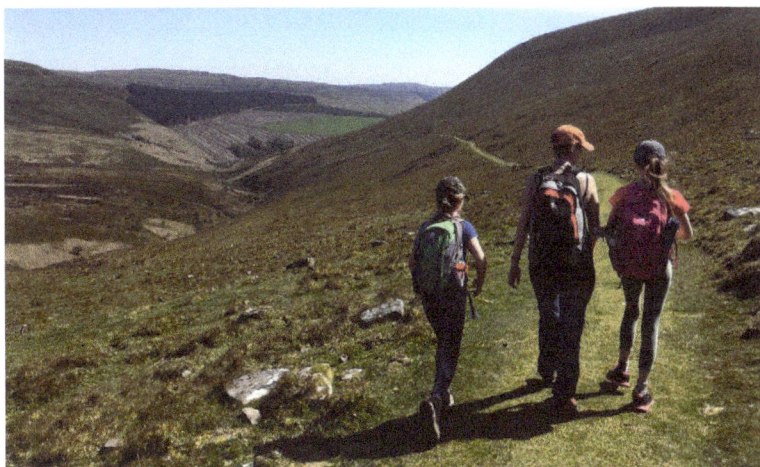

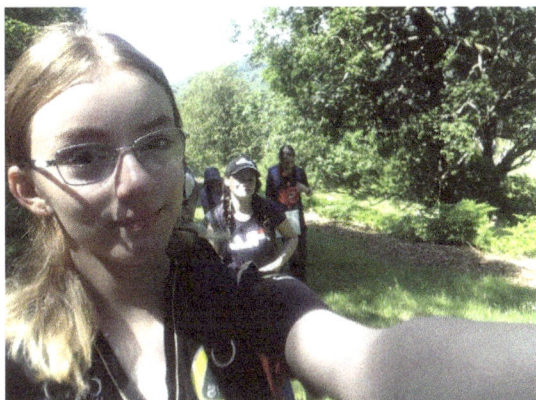

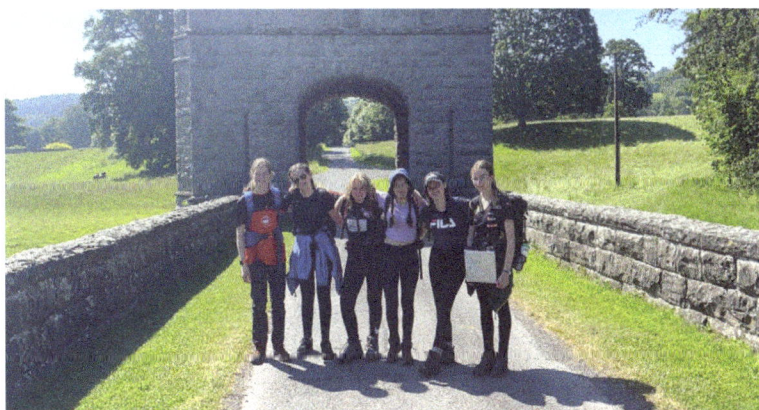

Walking with my family and friends.

Mummy's notes...

Background

Rosie was an amazing, beautiful, strong, and resilient young lady who tackled any challenge she faced in life with incredible strength and courage. She cared deeply for the people around her and would look after anyone who was lucky enough to know her. She was very quiet and unassuming, but this perhaps was where her phenomenal determination and iron will to fight what lay ahead, was masked.

Medically Rosie had contended with migraines over the years and had a brain MRI in June to rule out anything untoward. The MRI was clear and the cause of the migraines hereditary. That MRI was a fundamental trig point in the later diagnostic process.

At the beginning of July 2021 Rosie had Covid 19 but it only lasted a few days and she recovered quickly. We went on a walking holiday in Scotland afterwards and returned with Rosie then completing her four Duke of Edinburgh expeditions. She was so incredible with these challenges; she helped some of the other participants who were struggling to keep up. In late August she began to feel nauseous regularly and vomited every few days. We thought she was just exhausted and had over done it. This continued into September.

Dear Diary...

Blood Clot,

At the end of the day in school I got a cramp in my leg after PE, it was the most pain I've ever been in. My mum had to walk up to get me because the traffic was terrible. The pain in my leg was so bad at times my mum had to give me a piggyback down the road. When we got home, we took my socks off and my left foot was pale, white and freezing cold. I could not feel anything. The blood had stopped flowing to my foot it had also started to swell.

The pain moved up my left leg and lasted about four hours. We used a hot water bottle to get the swelling down and colour back into my foot. Mummy massaged my foot and leg to help the pain go away.

Later on we found out that the cramp would have most likely been a clot/thrombosis caused by a piece of my heart tumour breaking off and being pushed down my leg. I found out I have a narrow artery in my left leg and with the clot it had got stuck and caused all the pain.

19 September 2021

I am still finding it hard to walk long distances, but it is slowly getting better.

First hospital stay,

Up to now I have been vomiting every few days. We went to the GP a couple of times and tried some different medicines to try to stop it. These didn't work so when I went back a third time the GP had a listen to my chest and said she thought I may have A-typical pneumonia because she said she could hear something. She told us to go to the local hospital Emergency Assessment unit.

I was checked out by the Doctor and he said I haven't got pneumonia as couldn't hear anything, and because I'd had the cramp in my foot back in September told me to have a MRI scan. He thought it could be neurological. The scan showed little clots (emboli) on my brain that had not been there on the MRI I had back in June for my migraines. Another Doctor then came in and suggested I may need emotional support as thought I might have emotional difficulties making me sick. My mum and I knew this was not the case and something else was going on with me. The doctor said my heart was beating a bit fast, so because of the clots as well, they admitted me into hospital. They said they needed to find out where the clots in my brain had come from.

I was put onto a drip (IV) as they thought I was dehydrated and that was causing my heart to beat faster. My condition was getting worse by the day. Little did they know that all that fluid they were giving me through the IV was building up in my lungs because of the tumour, it was only making it worse.

They did an ECG, and said there was a little anomaly on it, but it wasn't anything to be worried about.

After six days they had run lots of the tests on me and still didn't know what was wrong. My arms were covered in bruises from the repeated blood draws and cannulas.

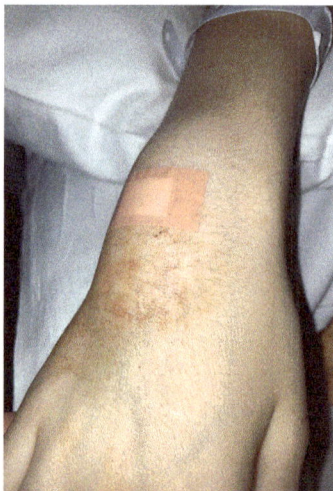

I had a reaction to a potassium drip and my wrist swelled up in minutes.

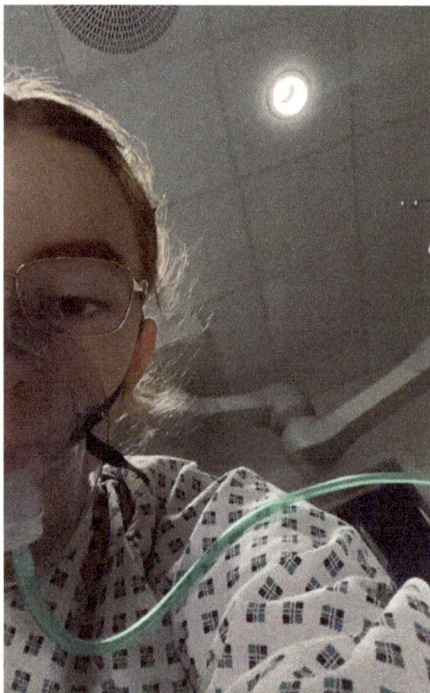

I had to have an oxygen mask on as was finding it harder to breath.

My blood oxygen level kept on dropping whenever I tried to sleep and there were gaps on the heart monitors where the electrical pulse in my heart had been stopping but they didn't know at the time. I am now sleeping fully upright because when I lay flat I can't breathe and the alarms keep going off. Every time I started to drift off to sleep, the alarms would go off again as my pulse and oxygen levels dropped. It was like torture, and I was so tired.

Each shift change there was a new doctor who wanted to do different tests on me. We didn't get much feedback on them before another doctor would then come in and do more. I think I had about 9 different doctors and at one point my mum said they couldn't do any more tests until they told me what the results were to the previous ones, and what the new ones were for.

Mummy's notes

After five days of no sleep and relentless tests Rosie was beyond exhausted. By day five/six she was unable to even tilt her upper body backwards and we had to prop her upright in the bed using the sofa cushions and every hospital pillow the wonderful nurses could help us find. She was struggling so much. We didn't know at the time, but it was due to the increasing volume of IV fluids being pushed back into her lungs from the heart tumour. Watching my little girl desperate to sleep but unable to because she was struggling to breathe and uncomfortable as she stated, was torture. I prayed for her to be able to close her eyes and rest but as soon as she started to drift off the alarms would piercingly blare out as her blood oxygen and pulse levels dropped to dangerous levels. I sat glued to the monitors watching every number and line.

The big surgery.

One of the last tests at our local hospital was an Echocardiogram (ECHO) on my heart. The female doctor clocked the tumour straight away and spent lots of time taking photos of the scans. It was that big she said I had to be operated on within 24 hours or I would not make it. This was life threatening. We were told it was a Myxoma and likely benign, not cancerous. Once the hospital and transport had been organised, at about 2.00am I was taken with my mum by ambulance to the Evelina Children's Hospital, London, part of Guys and St Thomas. My dad followed us behind in the car.

When we got there, we went into a glass walled treatment room which had lots of machines in it. They hooked me up to the machines and did another ECHO. We then met the cardiac surgeons who would do the operation. I was transported to theatre where they had to put in all the lines for the anaesthetic whilst I was awake, because I was a 'high anaesthetic risk'. I couldn't lean back at all at that point. They put a 12.5 cm central line in my femoral artery with me awake and no pain killers because of the time urgency. They normally do this after patients have gone to sleep, but they couldn't risk it due to the tumour in my heart.

The surgery was supposed to be five hours, but they had to repair the Mitral valve in my heart because the weight of the tumour had stretched it. The surgery ended up being seven hours 30 minutes. When it was over they took me to the PICU for recovery. My mum told me I was there for a couple of days and that even though I was heavily medicated, and couldn't even open my eyes, I would 'shoo' away the Doctors with my 'finger of dismissal'. She said they were all really impressed with the speed of my recovery.

I was then transported to Sky ward from PICU to continue recovering, which is the Cardiology (heart) ward for children.

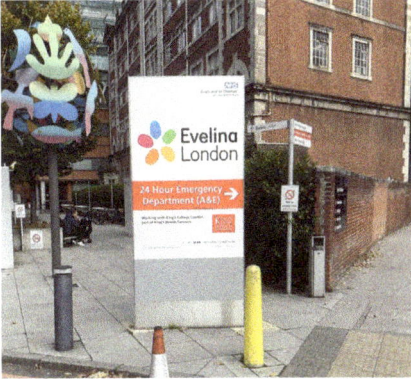

Figure 1, The Evelina London Children's Hospital where I had my open-heart surgery.

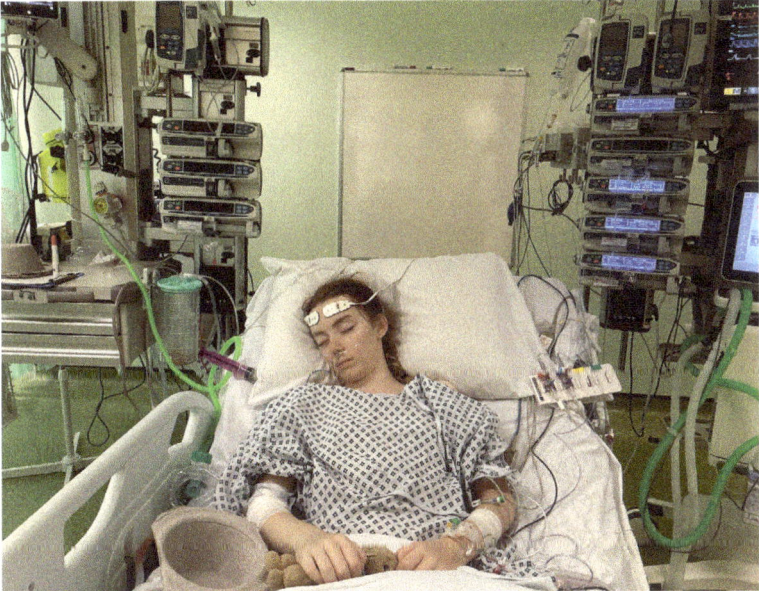

Figure 2, After surgery I was surrounded by loads of machines in PICU.

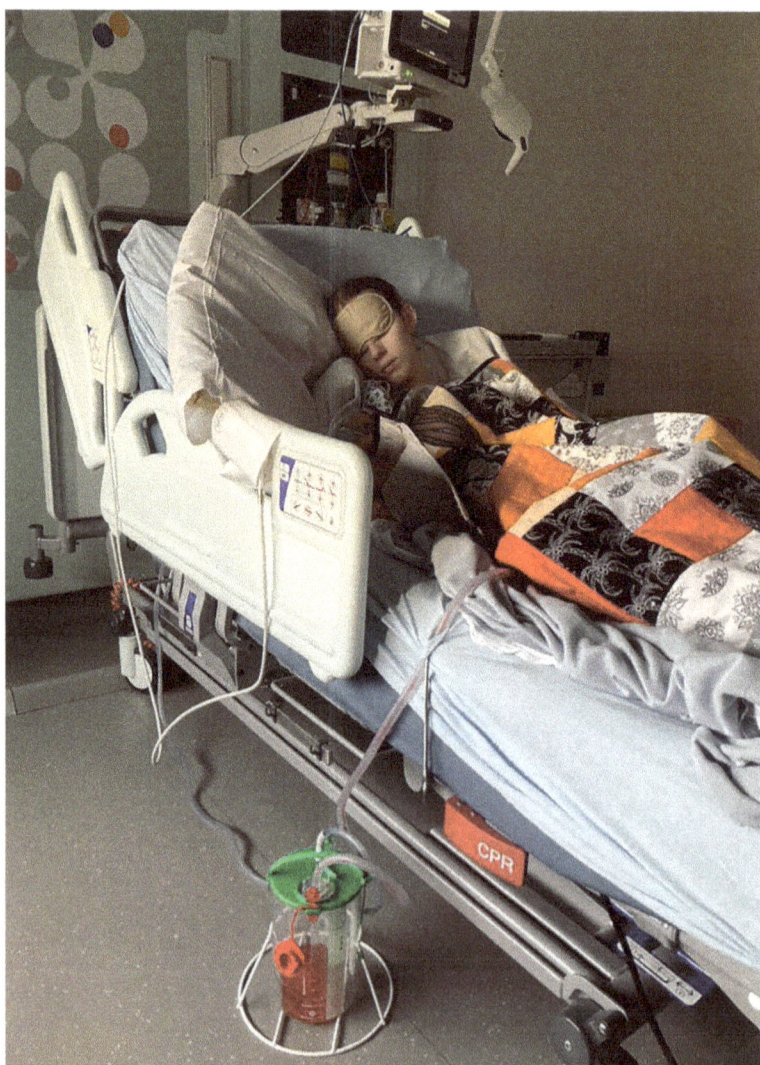

Figure 3, Recovering on the Sky ward still attached to a chest drain as I had a collapsed lung. The wonderful staff from PICU gave me a special handmade quilt made by volunteers in Project Linus UK. so I had something homely to wake up to. It is very special.

Mummy's notes

So humble. A testament of courage – pre op

Rosie's ECHO had been done at about 19:30pm in Wales, by late morning the next day our incredible girl was being prepared for surgery in London. I don't think we will ever meet anyone who showed as much courage as she did that night. Rosie must have been terrified and afraid of what was happening, but in her usual incredible way, she was calm, still trying to smile and said please and thank you even when she had blood drawn. After a tremendous amount of organising behind the scenes Rosie and I were loaded up on to the ambulance and daddy set up to follow in the car. Rosie later talked about the lovely 'WATCH' lady (paramedic) in the ambulance on the way down, who lent her phone and headphones so she could listen to music. The staff were all phenomenal, professional, kind and sensitive to her needs and dignity which was so important. We will be forever grateful to everyone who helped our Rosie.

We arrived in London and Rosie was taken into a large room loaded head to toe with machines and people buzzing around her like a hive around a Queen. Everyone had a role to play. I almost passed out and was guided into the side room. I realised along with not sleeping since Rosie was admitted almost a week prior, I'd not eaten for over 24 hours. One of her surgical consultants made me a cup of tea and toast, an act of kindness I was truly humbled by.

We will also never forget taking her into the crowded anaesthetic room, sat upright in the bed with everyone buzzing around to make sure our little girl would be okay. We held her whilst they had to insert her central lines fully conscious because she was such an immensely high anaesthetic risk. One in her forearm, but due to the multiple testing over the previous week it was hard to find a suitable vein, so I held her tight as they pulled the needle in and out trying to locate it. They then had to get the ultrasound to locate it visually, and they got it in the end. Once that one was complete it was the 12.5cm line that had to go into her inner thigh. They couldn't risk her falling asleep without everything in place as she was so critical. I didn't look at the needle at the time as was focused on holding her, trying to ease her pain but when they took it out later on, I was in awe.

Rosie's daddy and I then had to kiss her goodbye before surgery and then walked away. At that point these were the longest seven and a half hours of our lives.

A testament of courage – post op

As Rosie was heavily medicated and hooked up to all manner of machines after open heart surgery and being on bypass for seven hours 30 minutes she still continued to amaze not only us but the incredible PICU staff.

Rosie is a quiet young lady who would never want to upset or offend anyone. However, it was almost as if she had been on bypass and the blood that came back was full of 'sass!' Despite being unable to lift her eyelids open due to the medications and having a breathing tube in her mouth as well as chest drains, drips, and all manner of tubes and wires coming off her and connecting up to a multitude of machines, she still found a way of communicating which filled us with an enormous sense of relief and pride.

Rosie had stickers on her head to monitor brain activity and when these numbers/lines changed it indicated she was more conscious than sleeping. At this point her 'finger of dismissal' surfaced which she used to communicate to the doctor to go away! When she regained some control in her hand, with signing she also asked why she couldn't open her eyes, why the bed was moving (it was a special moving mattress to prevent pressure sores) and also "YOU'RE LEANING ON MY BREATHING TUBE!" I was mortified! There were so many tubes and wires around the bed it was hard to get close to her without leaning on something, but I was so elated to be told off by her!

Rosie then attempted to write even though she couldn't open her eyes or move anything but her right hand, by using a pen and white board. We answered her questions and, as she requested the breathing tube was taken out, it promptly was. As she became more conscious, she became aware of other patients in the room, including a very upset baby. Rosie's first spoken words were;

"STUPID BABIES!"

A testament of courage – "Stupid babies!"

This was so funny and out of character for Rosie as she wouldn't in a million years have said that had she not been in those circumstances. It is a funny anecdote she loved telling her friends and people in general about later on. We loved this post-op sass as it meant our Rosie was strong in herself and fully capable of tackling her recovery with intense determination. The nurses and doctors all enjoyed being told off or told to hurry up as it meant she was recovering well.

Those few post-op days were gruelling for Rosie as shortly after having open heart surgery, with three chest drains in and other tubes and wires she had to sit up and 'scoot' to the end of the bed. We were blessed with five amazing physiotherapists who helped her do this as it was a horrendous but imperative task for her to do for her recovery. She didn't want to do it as everything was so painful and uncomfortable, but she did. In fact, she was so outstandingly phenomenal with the progression of her physio, the following week when she had been on the Sky ward, the physios had walked in, seen her sat in the chair next to her bed and said "Oh, we're not needed now". They were blown away with her determination and perseverance through the pain.

Rosie had to have one of her chest drains in for a little longer than the others because she had a collapsed lung. This for her was probably the most frustrating aspect of her recovery at that time. She had to walk around carrying a little 'chest drain bucket' as well as her drip stand. However, in true Rosie style she cracked on, smiled and didn't let it stop her moving forward.

23rd October

Today I had my chest drain taken out, they put me on Buccal Diazepane which is a strong pain killer which caused me to go a bit giggly. I had my phone on me and started 'drunk/drug texting' my friends! My mum had to take my phone away and apologise to them!

1st November 2021

Diagnosed,

I can remember a lovely Doctor explaining to me that my tumour was actually malignant meaning cancerous. It is a very rare type of sarcoma. I felt very sad and didn't really know what to think. The good part though was that I would get to go home to Wales for further treatment, so I would be closer to my home and family.

Mummy's notes

After the monumental relief that our little girl had survived major open-heart surgery and had the tumour removed and mitral valve restructured, our lives then changed irreversibly.

We were called into 'the little room' to be delivered the horrendous news that the tumour we were advised was likely benign, was in fact malignant. It was so incredibly rare there are only 35 recorded cases of it in the whole world, only five of those children and Rosie makes it six. As this was so rare the next steps would need to be discussed at a national level with experts across the UK. As horrendous as it all was, we were confident with her treatment and were so grateful for the expertise and support within our NHS to ensure she was given the best possible chances.

Rosie often talked about "Doctor Tom" who broke the news to her that her tumour was cancerous. She spoke with fondness in how gentle he was when he explained it, and how hard it must have been for him to tell her. The humanity and kindness in the people who have helped her and made the most awful of things just that little bit more manageable, will be etched on our hearts.

Today my mum, dad and I went to the University Hospital Wales, Noah's ark for a cardio/oncology meeting. We were told I would need chemotherapy, the side effects of it as I would have to have some really nasty chemotherapy medicines, and that I would need six cycles, one every three weeks. They said I will probably lose my hair. I then had another ECHO on my heart and went home to prepare for the next phase. I was told they would do lots of tests before I start chemotherapy, as a baseline. As my tumour had been removed during the heart surgery, the chemotherapy was to make sure there were no new growths over the next few months of treatment.

8th November 2021

Today I had a PET CT scan so a full body scan and I was radioactive, so I had to try and avoid going near people for seven hours afterwards.

9th November 2021

First PICC line,

Today I am getting a PICC line put in my arm in the Teenage Cancer Trust (TCT) for chemotherapy. I was told treatment would start on the 12th.

Mummy's notes

The PICC line process is like a small operation you have whilst you're awake. Rosie had to lay down on her back whilst a guide wire was inserted through her upper arm and fed through the artery towards her heart. A machine was placed on her chest to ensure the guide wire was placed correctly. This then had a tube fed over it and secured at the point of insertion by little metal teeth just under the skin. On the outside of the skin are two 'ports' for access and on the inside, the securing 'teeth' and the tube to the heart through which the chemo and other medicines would be fed. The PICC line was a constant frustration for Rosie and staff because not only did it have to be inserted again shortly after it was initially done because it wouldn't work, but for every round of chemo, and bloods in-between it was touch and go whether one or the other ports would be blocked and usually entailed a 30 minute to one hour wait for an 'unblocker' medicine to work its magic before treatment or blood could be processed.

Rosie took these repetitive glitches in her stride and usually cracked some joke or other about it not working!

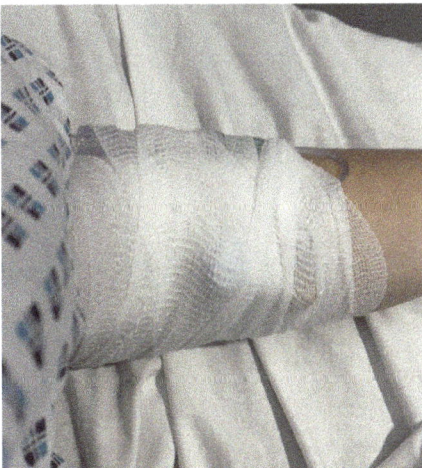

My PICC line which was bandaged up to keep it tidy and clean.

Today I had a full body MRI, ideally it would be six weeks after the operation but due to the urgency of needing the chemotherapy I had it three weeks after. It took an hour. I watched Jurassic World for the first part of the scan, but it was muted. When they turned the sound on for the second part of the scan it was in French!

I then went up to the ward and they said I had a small hernia at the bottom of my incision site, which is common after heart surgery (it went away on its own eventually). Then daddy and I got an iced coffee and stopped at Pizza Hut on the way home for pizza.

I had to get my PICC line taken out and put in again because the one they put in the first time didn't work and it needs to work for chemo.

First chemotherapy,

I had my first chemotherapy for the whole week. I slept for two days when we got home and then because I started getting a migraine, I took some oramorph. It didn't go well because it reacted with the chemo meds still in my system so I had to go in to hospital the next day. I then had to stay overnight for a few nights before I was allowed home again, so they could make sure I was okay.

Mummy's notes

Perpetual resilience…

The first chemotherapy was the worst as it took time to fine tune the anti-sickness medications. As Rosie had been nauseous and vomiting on and off since August it was tricky to work out the best medications, however it was eventually achieved. Rosie took it on the chin and dealt with it, never complaining, just working her way through the treatment bouncing back each time.

For chemotherapy Rosie would have her own room with a bathroom and a pull down bed for me to sleep on. Thanks to the incredible efforts of LATCH (the Welsh Children's charity) the process was made so much more bearable by their kindness. They provided food in a kitchen area as well as fridge space for families to store their own food, a microwave and other facilities to make being away from home just that little bit more manageable. They are without doubt a lifeline for families going through treatment and beyond. LATCH also have accommodation for parents should both want/need to stay, with one sleeping downstairs on the ward with their child and the other in a room upstairs which also had a kitchen, living room and washing facilities. As often was the case to be, the perpetual rush into hospital in between treatments due to infections/complications, self-care was the last thing you think of as a parent as the whole process is all encompassing in looking after your child. In our case it was also compounded by Covid-19 restrictions.

25th November 2021

The community nurse came to the house to change my PICC dressing. I didn't like it because my skin is really dry underneath it and it hurts. She took some bloods to check my neutrophils.

We met with some friends today in a café but I wasn't feeling very well and started shivering. We went home then mummy took me to hospital because my temperature was low. They took bloods and my gums were very sore and I have ulcers.

I have an infection as now have a high temperature, but I don't know what kind of infection it is. Because of the chemotherapy I'm neutropenic so had to isolate in hospital for 48 hours whilst on a drip of antibiotics. The infection could be my own body infecting itself because of the neutropenia. My hair has also started falling out and scalp is really sore and sensitive.

Still no cultures back from my bloods so they're not sure what the infection is.

I had to have an X-ray on my teeth to make sure I didn't have anything nasty in my gums that could be causing the infection. It was fun going through the underground corridors to the X-ray department. They're really creepy and it is where they filmed some of the Dr Who scenes.

2nd December 2021

Goodbye hair,

I had an ECHO on my heart, more bloods taken, and the dressing changed on my PICC line.

I've been discharged but before I left they had to give me a feeding tube because I've lost so much weight. This means I have to have a bottle of liquid feed on a little pump connected to a tube that goes through my nose and into my tummy.

When we got home we had to shave my hair off because it was all falling out and got really knotty. My scalp was also really sore.

I have another surgery on the 20th to remove one of my ovary's so I can have kids in the future. Chemo can damage your ovaries, so this was to protect one of them by taking it out and having it cryogenically frozen, in a place in Oxford. When I'm older, when I want children I know I have a healthy ovary to use if I have any difficulties.

My wig has also arrived from Little Princess Trust, it's beautiful. It is blonde, wavy and then it has blue underneath at the back.

6th December 2021

Back to hospital for the second round of chemo. Bloods taken and another head MRI. Chemo was a little better as I wasn't sick but still felt it. Home on Friday.

19

The headteacher from my school came round to see me today, it was awkward! Mummy, me and my sister have been watching The Hunger Games, it is really good.

16th December 2021

The nurse came to take bloods today.

Mummy's notes

20th December 2021 Rosie had her Ovarian harvest operation. She was in a lot of pain after the operation so spent an extra night on the ward to recover. This was followed by cardiology appointments, an MRI cardiac myocardial viability procedure (checking her heart function) and another ECHO. She took it all in her stride and was discharged a couple of days later.

23rd December 2021 The nurse came to the house to take bloods. Unfortunately, they ended up in the wrong lab which meant a trip to the hospital for another set to be taken on the 24th December. To make it easier we were allowed to go to our local hospital as it was closer. However, in true form Rosie's PICC line was blocked yet again which meant we then had to head to Cardiff main hospital after all to get it unblocked and bloods taken there.

My blood count is still too low, so the doctors have to push chemo again. Hopefully it will start on Friday 31st. I went to hospital for more bloods and for them to look at the sores in my mouth.

Chemo had to be delayed again because my neutrophils are still too low. They can't start it until my body has recovered a bit more. The nurse came and took more bloods so hopefully they will improve. I played with my sister on the laptops and Xbox all afternoon and evening.

In for chemo third round done. It wasn't as bad as the first chemo which was horrid as I kept vomiting. I think we're starting to get all the medicines right now to stop me feeling sick. Back home afterwards.

Woke up at 1:00am in the morning because I was constantly being sick and feeling nauseous and shivering so had to go to hospital in the middle of the night. I felt awful.

They put me on another drip of antibiotics for 48 hours, still waiting for more blood tests to come back. Once they came back I was allowed to go home on the 8th, yay!

Today I woke up got dressed and went to the hospital to have an ECHO scan. We watched Moana while the lovely lady was scanning me. We then went up to our usual ward and had bloods done. My PICC dressing was changed and we then went back home.

I played on the laptop with my sister and we got a takeaway.

I've been having regular blood tests at home in between chemo's to make sure my neutrophils were up enough to have treatment. Today I went to the hospital because I have a sore in my stomach and it's hard to eat or drink. I also have a little lump under my collar bone that has appeared. My neutrophils were too low so my chemo had to be delayed yet again.

Went back to the hospital again because the lump under my collar bone has got bigger. They gave me some tablets for my tummy pain.

I had a scan done on my kidneys to make sure I didn't have an infection.

The lump is sore so I had to have a scan on it. They think it's a cyst (infected under the skin) but I have to get it removed. They tried to drain it with a big needle whilst I was awake but it didn't work. I then had to have a surgery because it wasn't going down with all the antibiotics I was taking.

They finally let me have chemotherapy, fourth round done. Whilst I was in hospital my wheelchair has finally been delivered.

We went to see some puppies! We can't have one until my chemo has finished but I'm so excited. I was allowed to hold one of them and he opened his eyes for the first time ever. We will get a boy puppy and call him Argent after the character in Teen Wolf. We're getting him after my treatment is finished, I can't wait. The owners will hold on to him for us until we can have him.

Back to hospital and I had to have two blood transfusions.

Went to the hospital because we thought I had septicaemia. The ward was full so I had to go and stay on a general medicine ward to get yet another round of 48 hour antibiotics. They delayed chemo again to the 20th to give my neutrophils time to recover. I had to be given an injection of GCSF which helps boost neutrophils in order to try to keep the timings of my chemotherapy cycles. Chemo was delayed until 20th to give the injections time to work.

I got a camera from Dreams and Wishes, I'm so happy!! We had a KFC on the way home to celebrate.

Fifth round of chemo done and only one more to go. It's also now confirmed that I will need proton beam therapy which is a form of radiation therapy. This would have to be in Manchester as it's one of the only places in the UK that does it. A few years ago I would have been able to go abroad to have it, I would have enjoyed that!

We're going to Manchester tomorrow for my proton beam therapy assessment. This will be at the Christie hospital, Proton Beam therapy centre.

My pre-assessment for proton beam therapy,

We have arrived in our apartment and going to the proton beam centre for my clinic visit. They will change my PICC dressing there too. We went for a consultation with my doctor who told us what will happen during proton beam therapy and the side effects of treatment. He said I will be having 33 rounds of proton beam treatment which would take six and a half weeks. I wouldn't be allowed to go home until its finished.

We waited for a bit and then I had to have a special head mask made. The mask had to be moulded to my face and upper body for the treatment to make sure I didn't move at all. It was a bit tight, so they cut the eyes out as the pressure was horrible. My mum was giving me GCSF injections every day to try to boost my neutrophils and had to keep going until the doctor or nurse says to stop.

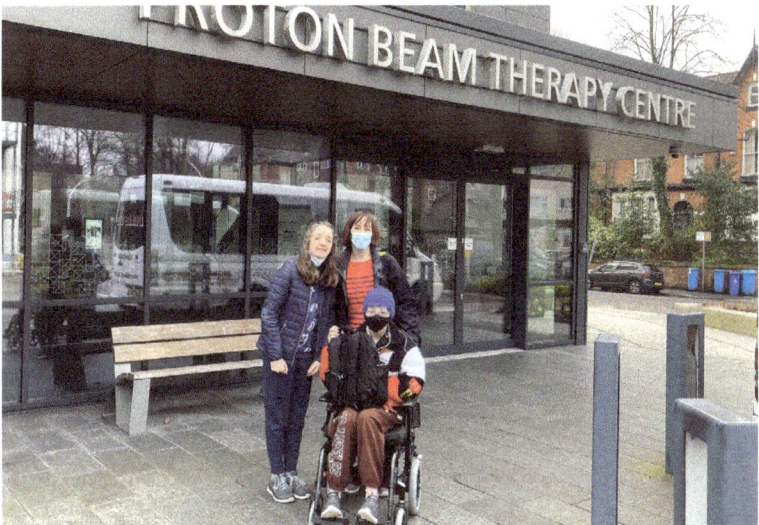

Outside the proton beam therapy centre, The Christie, Manchester.

25

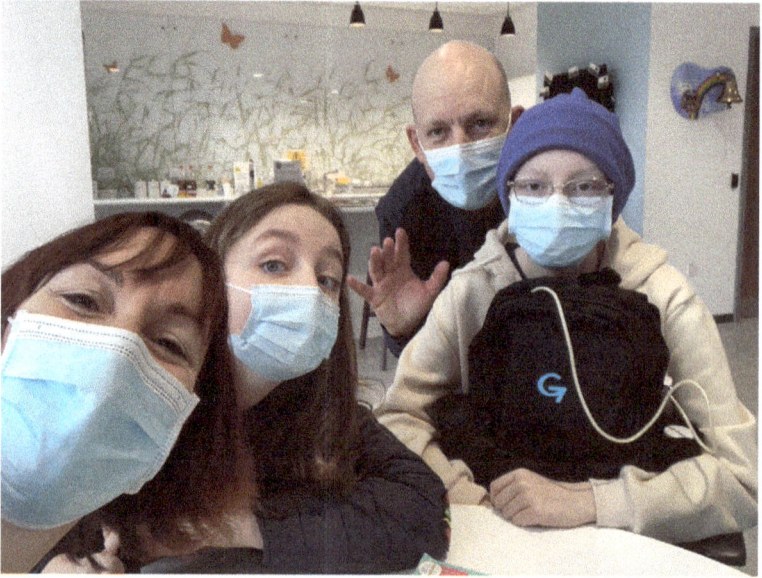

Inside the centre in the waiting area.

We went to the proton beam centre to have an MRI and CT scan. They gave me three permanent tattoo dots which were to help with getting me into the right position for my treatment. My left leg kept going numb but I kept on wiggling my feet which helped. Once all the bits were done at the hospital in preparation for the treatment, we went back to the apartment and started packing to go back home.

Saw the puppies and they had coloured collars on. We chose Argent who we'd also named 'Chunk' because he was the biggest and fluffiest. I put his new collar on him.

26

Today I went to get my kidneys tested in Noah's ark because the chemo medicines they are giving me are really strong. They need to make sure my kidneys are working like they should be. I was told it would take all day as they have to keep checking things.

We arrived at 9:00am and went straight to day beds, as usual my PICC was playing up, but the nurses eventually managed to get it working and took some bloods. We waited a bit for the doctor to come down and they then put a special dye in my PICC which made me radioactive. They would then take bloods at different times of the day to test if my kidneys were working okay.

Mum and I went to the concourse to get some food as were told we didn't need to be back up on the ward for a while. We then went back up to the ward and got some bloods done at 12:00, 1:10, 2:20 and 4:00. Once they did that, I went down to have another ECHO on my heart and we watched Despicable Me 2. I had a KFC on the way home.

14th March 2022
Monday

Last week of chemo,
Today we went to the hospital and to the radiology apartment for a CT scan on my heart. Then we went and I had an MRI on my head to make sure there are no clots in my brain where there were previously. We were later told the clots had gone which was good. I watched

27

Wonder Woman on the TV whilst I was in the MRI scan. They put a special contrast dye through my PICC line which makes the results clearer.

We then went to get some special papers so I could be allowed to access my medical scans and images to use for my book. After that we went upstairs to our ward and I had my feeding tube changed because it is only supposed to be in for three months and I've had it for five months.

Having my NG tube changed wasn't as bad as I thought it would be. It's usually the build-up which makes it harder than it is. I was admitted onto the ward ready for chemo and put onto anti-sickness meds ready to start chemo the next day.

17th March 2022
Thursday

Today is my last chemo bag on the drip stand and hopefully last night on the ward! The play ladies are making a sign for me saying 'well done Rosie' for tomorrow as I will be ringing the bell! We went to the playroom and saw Nico the therapy dog and had a chat then went back to our room. Unfortunately, my chemo bag was put up a bit late which meant I will be going home later tomorrow.

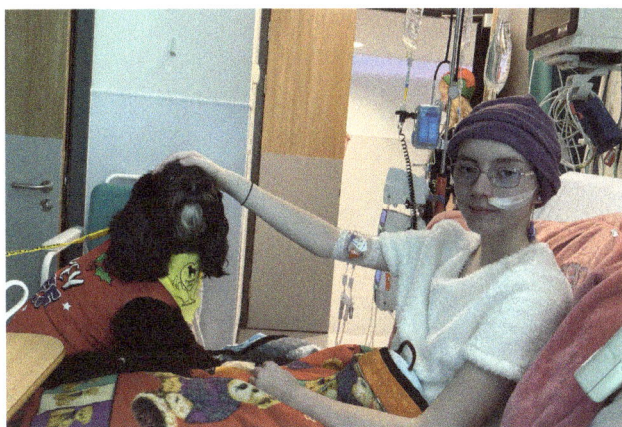

End of treatment,

Today is the day I am getting my PICC line taken out which I am really nervous about. My mum got me congratulations balloons which made me smile. I am only on fluids now to flush all the chemicals out my body, no more chemo bags!

It is 5:00pm and now is the time I was supposed to be ringing the bell, but my chemo was delayed yesterday pushing the time. Instead, they are only now taking my PICC line out of my arm. There were some complications with it so I had to have gas and air because the little metal claws that hold it in position under the skin were twisted and had got stuck. The nurse was amazing and worked so hard to try get it out. She had to cut the metal bits apart which wasn't nice and the whole process took an hour. After that my dad and sister were allowed to come in as I was a bit shaken up, and they sat with us so I could have a break.

Just after 6:00pm I was ready to ring the bell. The nurses and other patients and Doctors came out and clapped, it was very emotional. On the way home we stopped off for a KFC.

20th March 2022

Me and mummy went to see Argent and bought him his new toy 'Chad'. All the puppies loved him!

23rd March 2022

Today I had an MRI in preparation for baselining for Manchester. I had to have a cannula put in so the doctors could put a dye in for the scan. We didn't know where to go for that because our usual ward said not to go there. We were told to go to a different ward but they weren't expecting us. Then we were told go to yet another different one and when we got there, they didn't know where to put me.

So I went into the briefing room and waited. Eventually I had my cannula put in but the doctor forgot to take the tourniquet off, so I had blood running down my arm onto my new watch and onto my blanket. I then had my MRI scan on my heart, and it was very loud because they didn't put the headphones on me.

29th March 2022

Today we are going to Manchester for my proton beam therapy. My dad drove me and mummy to Manchester to help us settle in, then he left in the morning to go back home and look after my sister.

My first proton,

Today I had my first proton beam therapy, we went to the proton beam centre, and I had a quick clinic visit with the radiographer. The first proton therapy is always the longest because they have to do an x-ray and CT scan as well as a scan to make sure I am in the right position for the beams I have to wear the full-face mask for all of it, so my spine doesn't move.

We stopped after the first two scans because the camera broke and someone had to come in and fix it. Once that was fixed, I went back onto the table and had the mask put on and started my treatment. I had five beams in total all aiming at my heart. Then I got a star chart to record all my treatments, with pictures of my cats and Argent on it.

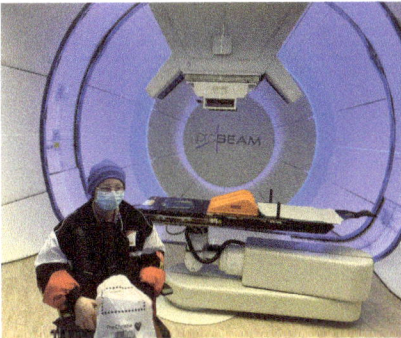

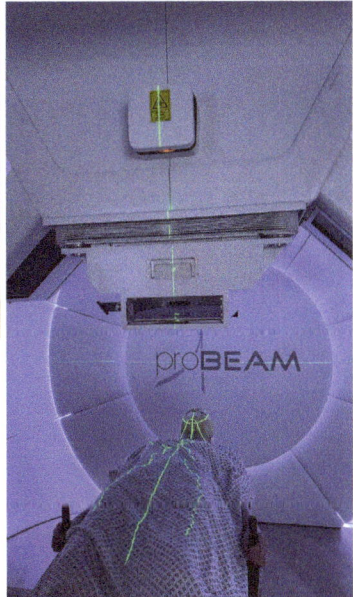

Proton Beam Machine

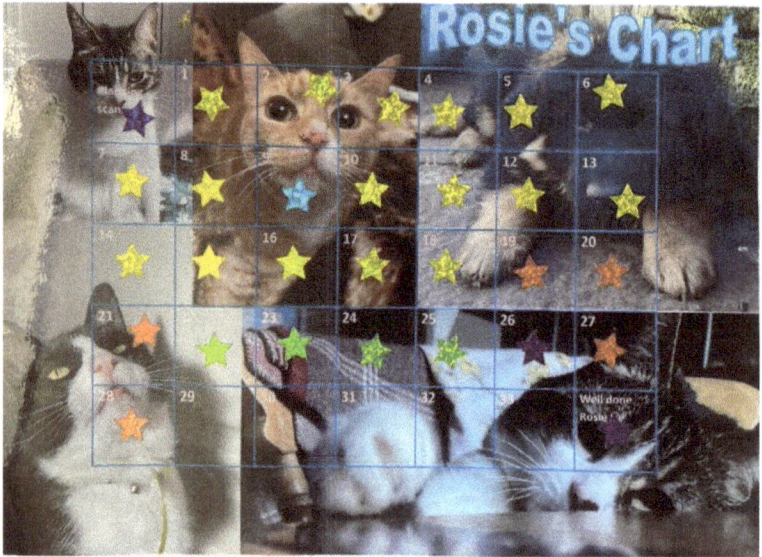

Star Chart

I had my second proton therapy today at 4:00pm so we had to wait a while because we caught the bus early. Didn't see the play worker today because there was only one and she was busy because the other play workers are on leave.

Today I had my third proton. We caught the 8:40am bus for my treatment at 9:30am but that was delayed a little, so whilst I was waiting, I had my bloods done then went in for my treatment. Mummy's been giving me injections every day since the end of chemo to boost my white blood cells so we are waiting to see if I can stop having them.

The results came back I am no longer neutropenic and can go off the pregnancy diet I was on for chemo (it's the same kind of diet) and I can stop the injections. This also means I would be able to have sushi for my birthday!

2nd April 2022

Today me and mummy went to the art museum which was a 12-minute walk from our apartment. Mum pushed me in my wheelchair and afterwards we went to a café. I had a cold Frappuccino.

6th April 2022

Today I had my treatment then we started our second bag of Beads of Courage [programme to support children through treatment] whilst we are in Manchester. I had already filled a bag with beads when I started the programme back in November. Then we went home to our apartment.

Today I had my seventh treatment and had bloods, and observations done as well as an ECG (ECHO cardiogram). We saw our consultant for the proton treatment he said that the gaps we were seeing on my Fitbit and in tests is most likely heart block, where the communication between the top and bottom of my heart is potentially stopping for a little bit.

Then I went and had my treatment and put a sticker on my chart.

Today my neck and shoulders were hurting whenever I lie down due to my mask, so the radiographers adjusted the mask. They cut out the eyes more and because I was also finding it hard to swallow because it pressed on my throat, they got a cigarette lighter and blew out a part under my neck.

They couldn't do anything about the back of my neck because they couldn't adjust the neck rest.

It's my birthday! We went on the proton bus and our new proton friends gave me a present! I had my treatment as usual; it was my eleventh round. The nurses and radiographers put a happy birthday banner on their doors, and when I went in the gantry for my treatment, they put the happy birthday song on. After that I put a sticker on my chart and got my beads, the nurses also made me a card and huge chocolate cake which was nice.

Mummy had booked us a table at a sushi restaurant to celebrate my birthday, so we invited our new proton friends who came, and we had fun.

14th April 2022

Daddy and my sister came up and we spent the evening in the Christie lounge with our new proton friends, eating pizza. The Teenage Cancer Trust had arranged for Dominoes to deliver pizzas to us on a Thursday evening. I didn't eat any as my tummy hurt but it was a fun chatting with them.

16th April 2022

We went to Primark to show my sister how big it is in Manchester. We brought some bits and pieces. Then daddy and my sister had to go home.

My tummy and spine is still really hurting, worse when I eat and drink, but pretty much all the time. I've not been able to swallow tablets or manage much of my tube feed. We took the Proton bus and saw one of the doctors. He gave me a stronger painkiller, then I went in for my treatment.

Today we had clinic and we finally saw my treatment plan. The beams are going through my spine and through my lower oesophagus and top of my stomach to get to my heart so that explains all the pain I've been having. My neutrophils have dropped to 1.2 but hopefully they will go up again. Then went and had my treatment.

Today I had my eighteenth treatment, there are three more weeks left until I'm free and I can go home! After treatment we went back to our accommodation and had pizza night up in the Christie lounge with our proton friends. One of my friends has done a time lapse of her proton beam therapy which I'd like to do too. When I see her next, I will ask if I can burrow her tripod to do it.

Today me and mummy went to an Alice in Wonderland themed tearoom, and it was really pretty. I didn't eat or drink anything as it was too painful, but it was good to get out. They do burlesque nights there, but mummy said it's for 18's and above. I walked for a bit and didn't use my wheelchair and when we got back mummy helped me with my book.

26th April 2022

Today was my twentieth treatment. My mask was sharp around the eyes from where the radiographers previously cut the eyes out, so they put tape round the edges. Then I went and did my beads and put a sticker on my chart. Angie from the Teenage Cancer Trust gave me a 'Gonk' which is a Gnome and it had a sparkly hat.

27th April 2022

Today I had treatment and then they put me on a longer lasting painkiller for my tummy. I went to the hospital school downstairs and printed off some of my scans so I can use them for my GCSE Art project.

1st May 2022

Today my dad and Molly my sister came up as a surprise but later I ended up being sick and my feeding tube came half out. My mum had to pull it out through my nose. She then called The Christie hospital hotline and they eventually said to go to the children's A&E as I had to have another tube put in straight away. They were worried I would get dehydrated as haven't been able to swallow to drink.

We waited and saw the oncology doctor to try and figure out what pain killer to give me because I am struggling to swallow and worried about how I would swallow the tube down. When they found something, it was a throat numbing spray it was horrible. It made my throat numb so I couldn't feel myself swallowing but it was also good because I couldn't feel the tube going down my throat, so I wasn't in so much pain.

2nd May 2022

Today I had my treatment. First off, we saw the nurses because my feeding tube had to be put in my other nostril yesterday, because the one it had been in before was too sore. Then I went in the moulding room with two radiographers to see if my mask needed adjusting because of the tube being on the other side, nothing needed to be done.

I then had my treatment and we're now counting down the days until I get to go home.

3rd May 2022

Throbbing hell,

Early morning at 1:40am I woke up with a horrid throbbing pain in my heart starting from the back of my head going down the left side of my body it lasted two minutes and it then started to pulse, which was also really painful. We thought it was a heart attack so was going to call an ambulance but then it stopped. We went in that day for my treatment as usual; the nurses and doctor checked me out and gave me the all clear.

5-7th May 2022

The same thing happened again in the night, with pain down my left side from my skull, down my left arm and side of my body. My left side felt a bit numb and sensitive. I had another weird spell with pain on my left side at about 10.30am and my heart rate went to 145bpm but then I felt okay. We met up with our friends later and had a fun time in the northern quarter in Manchester. Mummy pushed me in the wheelchair as I was tired but wanted to go out.

We then went to a cafe across the road from our apartment and I did a crossword on the menu. I walked across the road to get back to our apartment from the café and my heart rate went up to 170bpm which isn't good.

I rested on the sofa and felt a bit dizzy, but it passed. That evening I had a bath and I had one of the throbbing spells with intense pain from my head down my left side again. My left foot was physically pulsing I

39

couldn't control it, it wasn't nice. My heart was 65bpm.
I had some paracetamol, but I ended up throwing it up.

I had a clinic check-up and they think I might be
getting a severe reaction to the proton beams.

Today I threw up my medicine again and still can't
tolerate my feed. I was sick six times which isn't good
because I need to stay at a constant weight for my
treatment. I couldn't take any medications as I kept
being sick. We went to A&E and told them about the
pain I'd been having. They did an ECHO cardiogram and
an ECG and said I was fine.

Mummy's notes

9th & 10th May

*Rosie was on a multitude of medications almost every hour,
each one needed to go through her NG tube and then be
'flushed' with fluid. Due to immense stomach/lower throat
pain she was unable to tolerate much more than 5ml at a
time through her tube without it being agitated. She couldn't
physically eat or drink anything at this point. Her vomiting
had increased significantly even with anti-sickness
medications and the pain episodes she was experiencing on
her left side were debilitating for her. They also left her with
altered sensations on the left side of her body, sometimes
numb, sometimes super sensitive if she was touched.*

10th May 2021 *After another pain episode with her left foot
pulsating again in the night, I managed to record it on my
phone. We went to A&E again and she was eventually seen
by a neurologist. We explained Rosie's symptoms and
showed her the video of her pulsating foot. I also asked if it*

could be due to the emboli she had previously had in her brain. The neurologist examined Rosie and said that she couldn't see any obvious issues. She also stated that as the pulsating foot was not 'impactive' there was no real concern at this time. She said it was probably radiation related.

End of proton beam therapy,

Today we had a meeting with our consultant, and he said that because I've had the surgery, chemotherapy and most of the proton beam therapy I don't need to have any more treatment because I'm having a severe reaction. I've been to A&E three times now because of throwing up my feeding tube and the throbbing and pulsing pain on my left side, and I can't eat or drink at the moment.

I rang the bell that afternoon, and everyone came out to clap. Then I had to ring it again as mummy couldn't get her phone to record quick enough and hadn't managed to record it the first time! I was able to take my mask straight away which was good because you usually have to wait an hour for it after treatment due to it being radioactive. But because I didn't have my treatment today, I just got given it. Once I did all that we were allowed to go home!

13th May 2022

Coming home,

Today we are going back home, I'm so excited to see Lucy (my cat).

41

Today we picked up Argent the puppy!

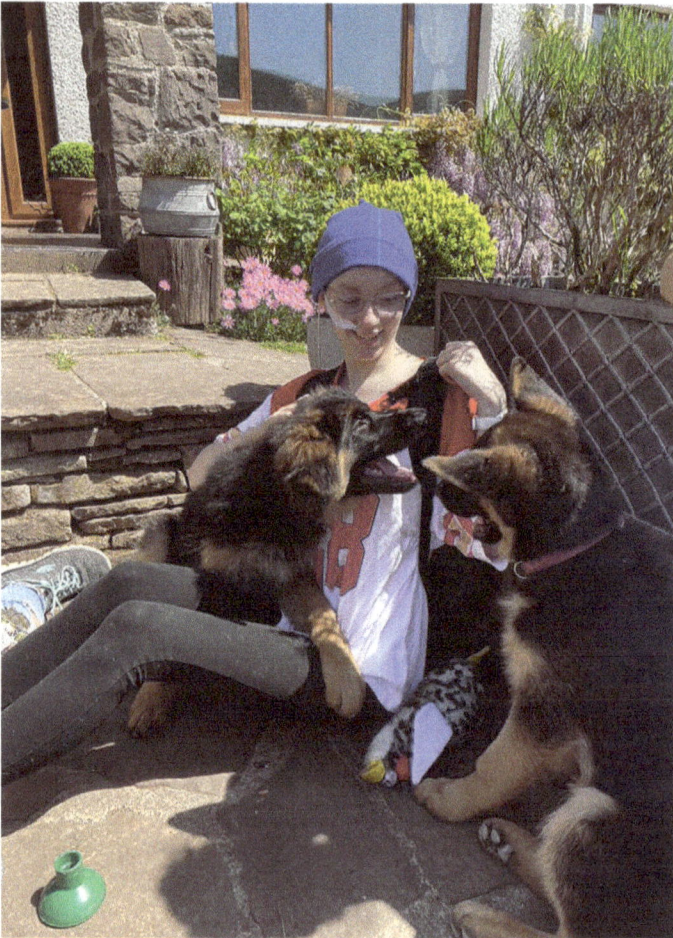

I've slept a lot. I am starting to tolerate my feed and had some strawberry milkshake. My tummy pain is getting a bit better but I'm still being sick.

As I've been sick so much and have a sore tummy, mummy phoned the hospital to ask if it was okay to give me re-hydration salts through my NG tube. The hospital insisted we come into Cardiff even though I didn't want to. I just want to be at home and rest. We had to wait for hours to see someone, and I was so tired and felt terrible after the journey. We finally got home at about 10.00pm.

18th May 2022

I spent a lot of the day sleeping. I'm still feeling sick but managing a little more fluid and a tiny bit of bread and butter. My left hand was pulsing in the bath this evening and then in the night my left leg went heavy and dead. My sock fell off and I couldn't feel my foot.

20th May 2022

Clinic in Cardiff today and I saw the dietician. Had a cardiac clinic too and my heart is okay. I had to stop halfway through my ECHO as my tummy was hurting, but we got it done.

21st May 2022

I am still feeling sick and had the throbbing pain again in my left side going to pins and needles. I had an aura when I went to bed, then in the night I had a horrendous headache, and the pain was unbearable. My mum thought it was a really severe migraine as we have a family history of them. By morning I had less and less control over my left arm and left leg, I was struggling to walk. I didn't want to go to hospital again, I've only just got home.

Mummy's notes...

Rosie was absolutely exhausted. She was recovering from nine months of gruelling cancer treatment, a severe reaction to the proton beam therapy and then the impromptu two hour round trip to Cardiff resulting in an extremely long day when she was running on vapours. Rosie needed to be at home, in her bed with no machines beeping or disruptions so she could begin to heal and recover. We were focusing on her rehabilitation as had been told in Manchester that the proton beam therapy was a curative treatment.

After what we thought had been a severe migraine on the 21st May, Rosie spent the next two days sleeping in bed. She struggled to co-ordinate her left arm and leg, but we felt the best place for her at that point in time was at home.

24th May 2022

I woke up and couldn't use my left hand side at all. My head was still really sore and I couldn't stop being sick. We phoned for an ambulance because I couldn't walk at all or use my left side.

We were transported to our local hospital where we saw the original doctor who had first treated me when I was admitted, before my heart tumour was diagnosed, which was nice. He said he saw my name on a list and wanted to come and say hi. He said he'd changed the way he diagnoses patients ever since he met me.

They put me through for an MRI because I couldn't feel my left side. I couldn't move my left arm or leg and was still being sick. When the results came through, they transported me and mummy to Cardiff hospital's oncology unit in an ambulance. One of our friends we'd made during my chemotherapy was on the ward and they gave us their room which was really nice.

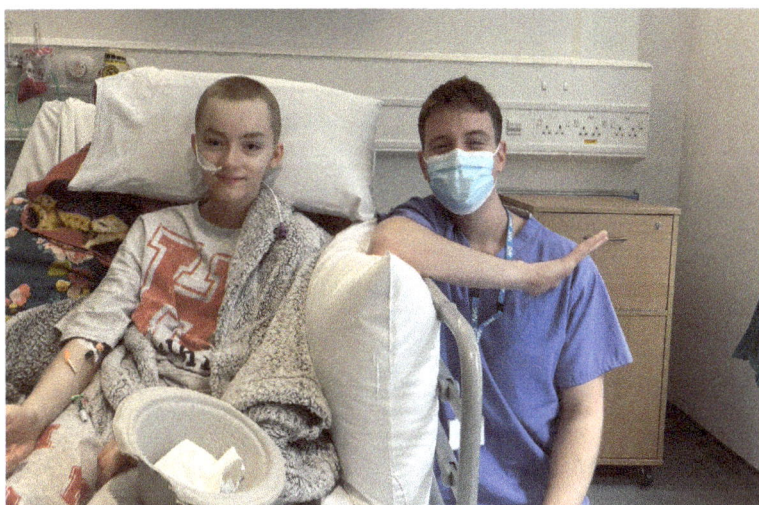

Me and Dr Dan

25th May 2022

2nd diagnosis,

Today we had a clinic meeting with our consultant. Whilst I was sleeping, they spoke to my mum and dad about the results of the MRI. After I woke up we went down for an ECG to check on my heart, but we had to do that quickly because I was still feeling nauseous, Then we saw the dietitian and went back up to our ward where I was told the results of my MRI.

It turns out that my cancer has come back but has moved to my brain and is too far in to operate on, there is nothing they can do about it. We don't know how long I have left to live because it has grown within six weeks and is aggressive. When she told me this the same questions went through my head like "how long have I got? What's going to happen next?", but I was too upset to ask. She said the best thing they can do is make me as comfortable as possible.

We got transported home and I got given a hospital bed to put in our living room because I can't walk. They also put a syringe driver in my leg so I can have some stronger medicines at home, a community nurse will come over every day to refill the driver.

Nana and Gramps were there when I got home, they gave me a cuddle (Nana and Gramps are my mum's mum and dad).

29th May 2022

Bampa and Glasses (my dad's mum and dad) came over and we signed the Jarman family bible. It was fun.

30th May 2022

The doctors had prescribed me with steroids to reduce the swelling in my brain. The tumour is pressing on a nerve causing my arm and leg to twitch and I can't control it. It is causing me a lot of pain. The steroids make me feel really hungry. For breakfast I've had a salmon bagel and a bacon sandwich.

Mummy's notes

We have two main downstairs rooms in our house connected by a long hallway. In the living room we had Rosie's hospital bed, standing frame and other equipment so we could care for her at home. Rosie's sister put photos up of all her friends and family and we made it as special for her as we could.

In the kitchen the work surface was piled high with multiple medications and equipment needed to facilitate her care at home. My phone had 14 different alarms on it to ensure I remembered to administer the multitude of medications she needed.

Rosie's cat Lucy stayed with her nearly all the time, apart from when Argent the puppy was in the room.

As the steroids, new painkillers and anti-sickness medications began to take effect Rosie began to eat more. She became perkier and more determined to make the most of every minute she had. Her tummy pain had subsided, and she began to enjoy food again for the first time in almost a year.

Rosie made multiple lists of tasks to do, mainly involving art given she was limited with left side paralysis, and we were grateful to do everything we could to get her what she needed.

Rosie didn't complain or dwell, she just wanted to keep busy.

Today I was supposed to fly in a Merlin helicopter from 845 Naval Air squadron and Commando Helicopter Force at 10,000 feet which my Uncle Simon had organised, but I'm too ill so he organised for one to fly over our house instead. We managed to get my wheelchair outside and we waved at the pilots as they circled the house instead! They gave me a framed picture of all the people it took to make it happen.

7th June 2022

Today I rode in a Lamborghini with a racing driver called Rory Collingbourne, it was so much fun. We got pulled over by the police, too! It was organised by a charity called Dreams and Wishes.

8th June 2022

Today I rode in a helicopter, and it was a total surprise. I was having another drive in the Lamborghini, and we pulled up in an airfield. I sat in the front with mum in the back and we flew over our town.

15th June 2022

Today we went to Trago mills and mum had arranged for us to be allowed to take Argent in with us. We got lots of art stuff to keep me occupied and then I had a sausage roll, cream tea and candy floss.

Today I flew a Plane! It was terrifying as I could only use my right hand but fun. Dreams and Wishes had organised it for me because I want to be a pilot. When we got home I did some more work on my book.

17th June 2022

Today I drew on a mini canvas and finished a photo book I've been working on. We managed to get the wheelchair into the kitchen so I could have a change of scene and I made some coconut bites with my sister.

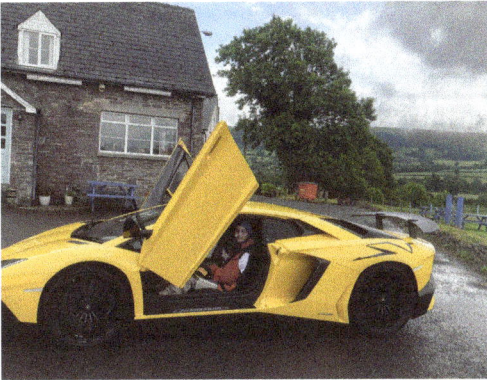

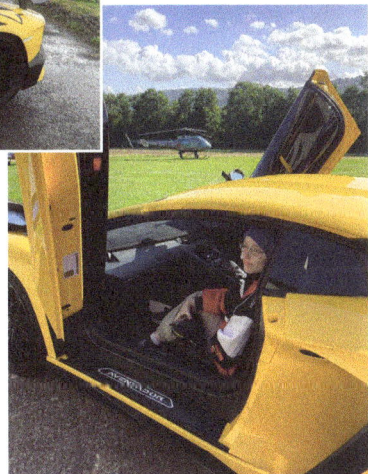

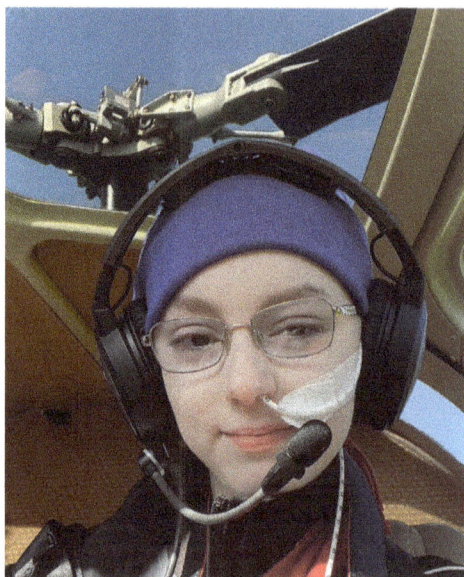

Thank you

DREAMS&WISHES

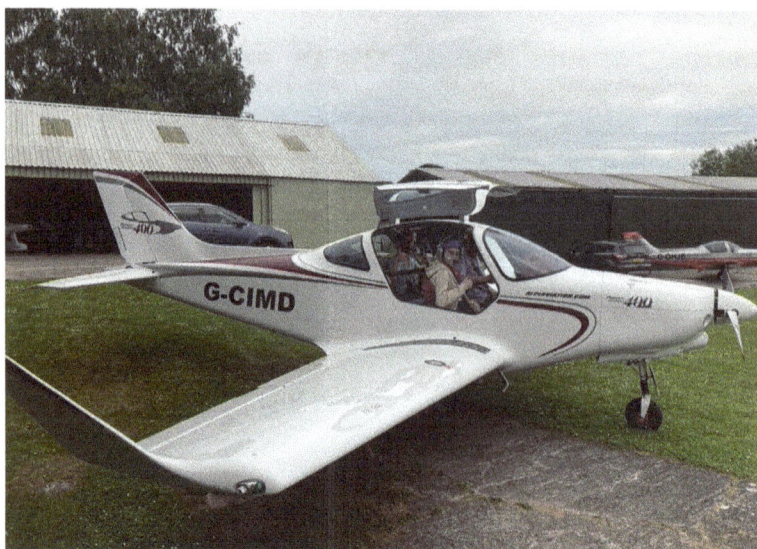

Father's Day

Rosie wanted us to have a special meal at the local hotel to celebrate Father's Day and we managed to book a table there with wheelchair access. We arrived in good spirits, settled at a lovely table by the window and ordered our food.

Unfortunately, Rosie had begun some stronger medication at this point due to increased pain and became very unwell with it. She felt so poorly and could barely keep her eyes open. She reluctantly agreed to let us take her home. We then changed her to a different medication, and she picked up again after a long sleep.

Rosie was now sleeping until about midday on most days and getting increasingly tired. One of us would always be sat in the living room with her to keep her company and be there if she needed anything. Lucy always curled up on her blankets. When she woke she would want to be doing something so would go into her wheelchair so we could take her into the kitchen or outside.

20th June 2022

Today I found out that through our lovely proton family a charity in a remote village in Uganda has heard about me and donated a water tank to a 90-year-old man, in my name. They sent a video of the village children singing 'Thank you Rosie Jarman'.

The pain doctor came to see me today.

My friends are now allowed to go into town for lunch and they all came over to see me today. It was fun.

Mummy's notes

24th June was Rosie's last diary entry. Having her friends around on that Friday meant the world to her and us.

25th June – Rosie made some biscuits in the kitchen with her sister and decorated them ready for Bampa and Glasses to visit the next day. We had to cancel the visit.

Our amazing, beautiful, courageous 15-year-old daughter Rosie finally passed away at 8.00am on 27th June 2022.

Sometimes the bridges that are hardest to cross

Lead to the most magical places

Sarcomas

Sarcomas account for approximately 15–20 percent of cancers in children and young adults (this is compared to 1 percent of all adult cancers).[1] Sarcomas can occur almost anywhere in the body but common sites are the head and neck area, genitourinary tract and limbs.

There are two main types of sarcoma: soft tissue sarcoma and bone sarcoma. Soft tissue sarcoma, often referred to as STS, develops in the soft connective tissue such as the muscles, cartilage, tendons, or fat. Bone sarcoma forms in new tissue in growing bones. Within the two main types of sarcoma, there are more than 70 subtypes based on the origin and location of cancer.

The most commonly diagnosed types in children include[2]:

Ewing Sarcoma: A rare type of childhood sarcoma that grows in bone or the soft tissue surrounding it. It is typically found in the centre of the body, such as the chest, pelvis, or vertebrae, but can appear in any bone. It is most often diagnosed during puberty, but can also occur in younger children or adults.

Rhabdomyosarcoma: This is the most common type of childhood soft tissue sarcoma and accounts for nearly 5 per cent of childhood cancers. It develops in the skeletal muscles. Though it can affect anyone, it primarily occurs in children under four years of age.

Osteosarcoma: This type of sarcoma typically originates in the 'long bones' of the body, such as the bones of the arms and legs. It is the most common type of bone cancer in children and is usually diagnosed during puberty or times of growth spurts.

Other types of sarcoma include:

- **Fibrosarcoma** – develops in fibrous tissue
- **Synovial sarcoma** – develops in cells near the tendons and joints
- **Liposarcoma** – develops in fatty tissue
- **Angiosarcoma** – develops in the inner lining of blood vessels
- **Chondrosarcoma** – develops in cartilage

Causes of childhood sarcoma

It is not yet fully understood why sarcoma develops in an individual person. Some factors may increase the risk of developing a sarcoma. These include:

- Genetic disorders such as neurofibromatosis and Li-Fraumeni syndrome
- Viral infections (e.g., glandular fever or HIV)
- Prenatal genetic changes caused by chromosome abnormalities
- Exposure to certain chemicals, such as vinyl chloride
- Previous radiation treatment (e.g. radiotherapy)

Common symptoms include:

These symptoms may vary greatly depending on the sarcoma and its location.

- Most cases people will have a lump in some part of the body
- The lump can be painful
- Abdominal pain
- Cough
- Breathlessness
- Vomiting

Staging

Before treatment for sarcoma can start, staging is required. This usually involves scans (such as CT, MRI and PET scans) and will inform doctors whether the sarcoma has spread to surrounding structures near to the primary tumour and whether it has spread to other parts of the body. Although doctors use complicated 'staging systems' to describe sarcomas they generally fall into the following groups:

- **Localised (non-metastatic sarcoma)** The cancer is confined to one place and has not spread to other parts of the body. It may have been biopsied or partially removed by surgery.
- **Sarcoma with loco-regional spread** The cancer has invaded or spread to nearby structures such as lymph nodes but there is no sign of it in organs distant from the primary tumour.
- **Metastatic sarcoma** The cancer has spread from where it started to other parts of the body.
- **Recurrent sarcoma** The cancer has come back (recurred) after it has been treated. It may recur in the original location or in another part of the body.

Treatments include:

- Surgery
- Chemotherapy
- Radiotherapy
- Proton beam therapy

Treatment side effects

Everyone gets different side effects with what treatment they're having. The most common ones are:

Surgery

- Scar
- Possible collapsed lung
- Sore throat (from breathing tube)
- Hernia
- Might have to learn to walk and talk

Chemotherapy

- Nausea/sickness
- Hot flushes
- Hair loss
- Low blood counts (neutropenia)
- Fatigue/tiredness
- Loss/gain of appetite
- Loss/gain of weight
- Skin/nail changes
- Neuropathy (numb/sensitive/tingling hands/feet)
- Bowel changes
- Fertility changes
- Change in taste

Proton beam/Radiotherapy

- Redness/soreness around treated area
- Tiredness/fatigue
- Sore throat
- Difficulty swallowing
- Shortness of breath
- Nausea/sickness

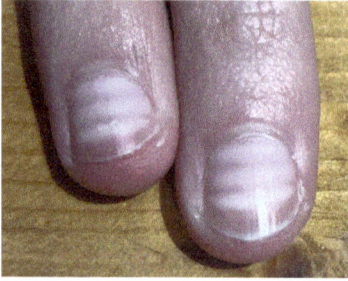

Figure 4, Chemo Nails

Figure 5, Hair loss, and nasogastric feeding tube due to nausea/sickness and loss of appetite.

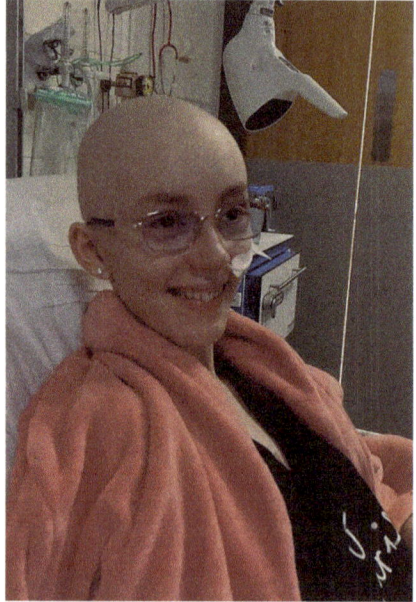

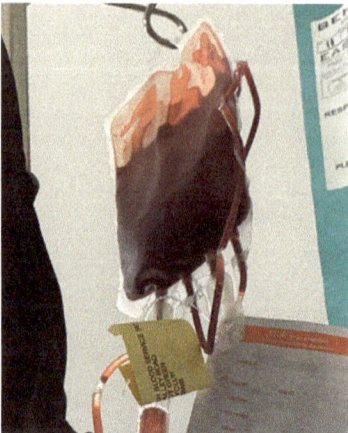

Figure 6, Blood transfusion due to low blood counts and anaemia.

Long term

Depending on where your being treated it may vary.

- Skin changes
- Secondary cancers
- Can affect your fertility
- Tiredness
- Heart problems

After having HGUPS (long term effects)

- High heart rate
- Dizzy spells
- Might have heart problems
- Possible spread of the sarcoma

Survival outcomes

Survival rates for children's cancers have improved significantly over the past few decades and overall survival rates are around 85 percent for all cancer types. Unfortunately for sarcomas there has been little overall improvement and survival rates remain lower than for many other cancer types such as leukaemia and lymphomas. Overall, approximately 65–70 percent of children with sarcoma will be cured[3], but this could be lower or higher and is influenced by several factors including tumour size and location, type of sarcoma, the age and overall health of the child at the time of diagnosis and the response to treatment.

My Cancer

Cardiac tumours

Primary cardiac tumours (tumours originating from the heart are very rare). Most (75 percent) of cardiac tumours are benign with the commonest type being myxomas which usually occur in the top two chambers of the heart (atria). The commonest primary cardiac tumour in childhood is a rhabdomyoma which are often associated with genetic conditions such as tuberous sclerosis. Other rare tumours such as fibromas, haemangiomas and lipomas can also occur in the heart.

Malignant cardiac sarcomas are very rare, with around one in every thousand soft tissue sarcomas arising from the heart.[4]

Cardiac tumours usually present with symptoms of cardiac failure (e.g. breathlessness, unexplained loss of consciousness, chest pain) or symptoms of ischaemia or infarction because of embolization of tumour or blood clots to the brain and other parts of the body. In the early stages cardiac tumours can be difficult to diagnose because the symptoms are very similar to those caused by more common conditions.

Treatment for cardiac tumours is complicated and usually involves surgery with or without further treatments including chemotherapy, radiotherapy or proton beam therapy.

High Grade Undifferentiated Pleomorphic Sarcoma (HGUPS)

This specific type of sarcoma is a soft tissue sarcoma and is found in the heart and is very rare, mostly found in adults but still rare and even rarer in children. There are only thirty-five other recorded cases in the world and only five of these were children. If not treated quickly this sarcoma is fatal.

Unfortunately, it is the type which can spread quickly and is very aggressive.

Symptoms include:

- Constant nausea/constantly vomiting
- Breathlessness
- Dizziness
- High heart rate
- Constantly clearing your throat/coughing
- Sleeping raised
- Blood clots
- Cough
- Paralysis
- Uncontrollable throbbing/pulsing

My Treatment Plan:

Surgery

Seven and a half hour open heart surgery to remove the primary tumour and repair damage to the mitral valve.

- From initial admission at our local hospital to discharge from the Evelina London Children's Hospital this took just under three weeks.

Chemotherapy

Chemical drug therapy containing cytotoxic (anti-cancer) drugs, designed to locate and destroy cancer cells.

- Six rounds of chemotherapy on a three-weekly cycle. *Due to complications, infections, transfusions, two small operations due to further chemo related complications, multiple emergency admissions for infections, etc., this took around four months.*

Proton beam therapy

Laser beam therapy where they use lasers to destroy the remaining of the cancer cells.

- 33 rounds of proton beam therapy however this was reduced to 28 rounds due to complications. *This took around six weeks.*

Emergency admission due to left side paralysis

- Two nights for reassessment and then return home for palliative care.

My heart scan

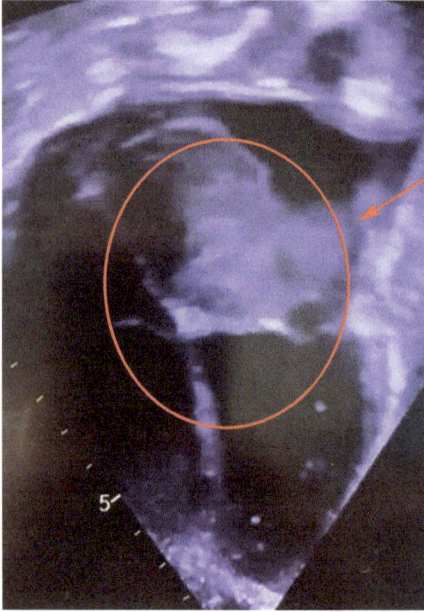

15cm tumour in the left atrium of the heart.

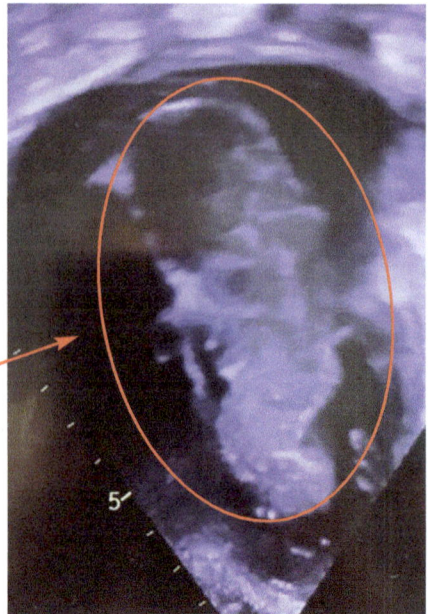

Tumour going in the left ventricle, causing the valve to stretch and lungs fill up with fluid.

My brain scan

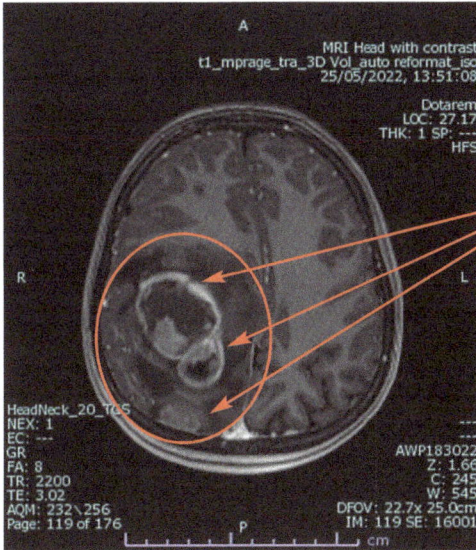

Three tumours that had embolized to the brain from the primary tumour causing substantial swelling.

Chemo Tips

Use moisturiser

Your skin will get really dry cause of the meds.

Stay hydrated

You need to flush all the meds through your body or it can cause problems.

Bring activities

You never know how long you'll be admitted for.

Take your anti-sickness tablets regularly

Wear chemo practical clothing

You don't want to be trapped in hospital with uncomfortable clothing.

Shower or bath pre chemo

You might feel too tired the next day.

Your taste will change

Be prepared you might lose your hair

Lots of people shave their hair at the first sign of loss (that's what I did) but it's up to you.

Always take a blanket or a duvet if you're allowed

Some nights can get cold in hospital, and they can run out of blankets.

Sleep lots

You won't get much sleep in hospital, so get as much as you can when you're at home.

Stay in contact with your friends

You might not feel like it but it's always good to have someone to talk to.

Take care of your dental care

You might not feel like getting up every day to do your teeth but you must keep on top of it. You can get a cup and do it in bed if you're not feeling like getting up.

Hospital Packing List

Cosmetics

Try and use non fragrance products, as your skin will become very sensitive due to chemo.

- [ ] Lip balm
- [ ] Hand cream
- [ ] Face/body moisturiser
- [ ] Sun cream
- [ ] Body wipes
- [ ] Natural deodorant
- [ ] Baby shampoo
- [ ] Baby toothbrush (you might get sensitive gums

Clothing and accessories

Whatever PICC or central line you have depends on what you wear, because that will need to be accessed when you're having treatment.

- [ ] Short sleeve tops/t-shirts
- [ ] Sweatpants
- [ ] Leggings
- [ ] Short sleeve pyjamas
- [ ] Baggy jumpers
- [ ] Slippers
- [ ] Warm blanket
- [ ] Comfy cushion
- [ ] Comfy underwear
- [ ] Dressing gown
- [ ] Warm/ comfy socks
- [ ] PICC line covers
- [ ] Eye mask
- [ ] Hats (I recommend beanies)
- [ ] Toiletries

Objects

- ☐ Earphones
- ☐ Ear plugs
- ☐ Mini fan
- ☐ Scrapbook
- ☐ Activity books
- ☐ Calendar
- ☐ Phone chargers
- ☐ Magazines/books
- ☐ iPad/laptop
- ☐ Diary

For Parents/Carers

Most parents/carers forget about themselves and forget what they need. Some might not eat for days cause their busy worrying about their child.

- ☐ Flask
- ☐ Food
- ☐ Blanket
- ☐ Note pad
- ☐ Comfy clothes
- ☐ Folder
- ☐ Activities
- ☐ Eye mask
- ☐ Spare underwear
- ☐ Toiletries
- ☐ Medicines

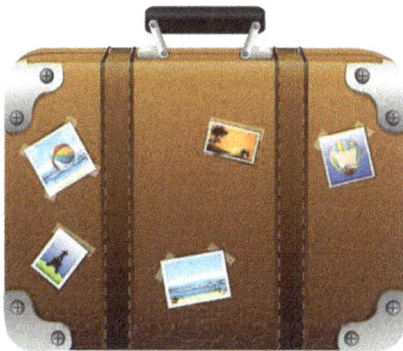

Thrombosis

The formation or presence of a blood clot in a blood vessel. The vessel may be any vein or artery.

I had a thrombosis in my left leg because of my heart tumour squirting out clots and that I have a narrowing in one of my arteries which made the likely hood of getting a thrombosis higher.

Symptoms:

- Swelling in leg
- Pain in leg
- Red or discolouring in the skin
- Unusual temperature in the leg

My symptoms with a narrowing artery and the clot:

- Pain in my leg
- Couldn't walk
- Swollen foot
- Limited circulation
- Very slow capillary refill
- Pale white leg
- Numbness moving up my leg
- Pain lasted roughly four hours but may vary

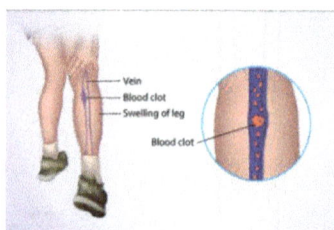

Treatments:

- Blood thinning medicine
- Catheters to widen affected vessels/arteries
- Hot water bottle

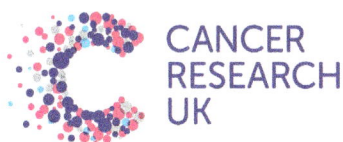

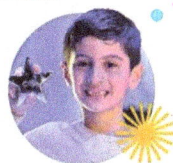

Cancer Research Star Awards

Recognise your child's courage in facing cancer by nominating them for a Star Award. The awards are open to all children under 18 who live in the UK and have been treated for cancer within the past five years.

It is run by Cancer Research UK and given to children undergoing chemotherapy.

Partnership with:

- TK Maxx
- Emma Thompson
- Phil Gallagher
- Aston Merrygold

And more…

TK Maxx sponsors the Star Awards scheme, which recognises the strength of children and young people across the UK who have been diagnosed with cancer.

They have been supporting Cancer Research UK since 2004 and is the biggest corporate supporter of research into children's and young people's cancers for the charity.

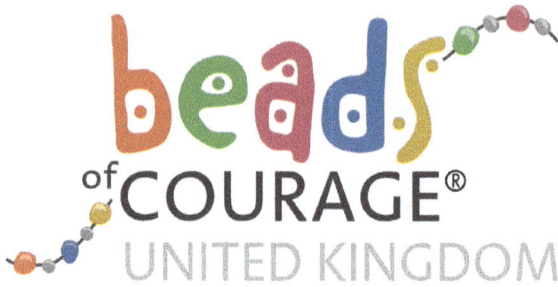

Beads of Courage

Beads of Courage, also known as Be Child Cancer aware, helps children RECORD, TELL and OWN their stories of courage during treatment for cancer and other serious life-threatening illness.

It was set up in 2004 by three families with a child with a cancer diagnosis.

Every Bead has a specific meaning here are a few:

- **Black** Pokes (blood taken etc.)
- **Yellow** Hospital stays
- **Red** Blood transfusion

Benefits:

- Helps to decrease illness-related stress.
- Increase the use of positive coping strategies.
- Restores a sense of self.
- Takes your mind off the illness for a little bit and distracts you.

More tubes than human

Having more tubes and drains in you isn't as fun as it may seem, these pages are going to tell you the tubes and drains you might experience having after heart surgery and during treatment.

Before/After Surgery

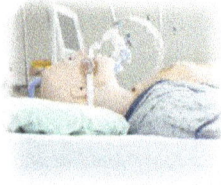

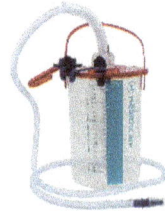

Breathing tube

Is a tube which helps you breath if you are put under anaesthetics for surgery.

They are usually removed but if the patient is finding it hard to breath or are seriously ill they will keep it in for a bit longer.

Advantages:

- Helps you breath
- Keeps you alive under anaesthetic

Disadvantages:

- Sore throat after it is removed
- Can't speak when it's in

Chest drain

It is inserted through the chest wall to drain any unwanted fluid, air, blood, etc.

Advantages:

- Removes unwanted substances
- Easier and less painful to remove the substances

Disadvantages:

- Hard to sleep on your side
- Have to carry the drain around

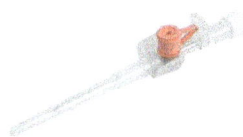

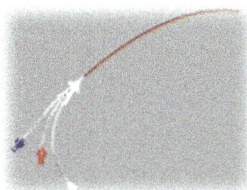

Cannula

Is a thin tube inserted into a vein or body cavity to give medication, drain off fluid or take samples of blood.

You will have lots of cannulas in your hands and arms.

Advantages:

- You don't get stabbed as often for taking blood

Disadvantage:

- They can get agitated if put in wonky

Central line

These are catheters placed in a large central vein in the neck, arm, femoral, or chest, which they use to put medicine down.

If you are having heart surgery you would have three – one in your arm, one in your femoral and one in your neck.

Advantages:

- Delivers medicine right into your bloodstream
- Gives medicine quickly

Disadvantages:

- Can damage your veins if not placed correctly
- Risk of infection

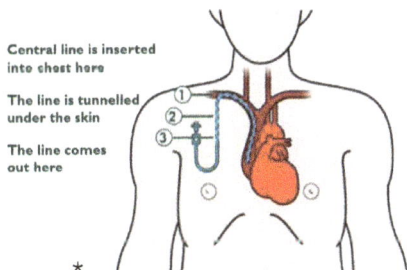

Central line is inserted into chest here

The line is tunnelled under the skin

The line comes out here

*

* Original illustration developed by Macmillan Cancer Support and used with permission.

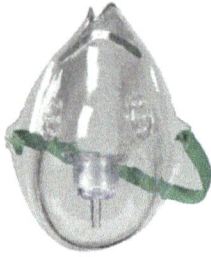

Oxygen mask

An oxygen mask transfers breathing oxygen gas from a storage tank to the lungs, which helps you breathe if you need it.

Advantages:

- Helps you breath
- Gives you oxygen

Disadvantages:

- You can't talk
- Claustrophobic

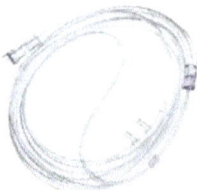

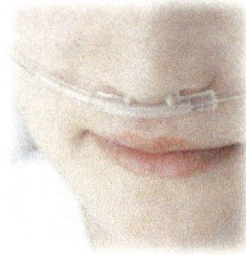

Oxygen nasal cannula

This is a device used to deliver supplemental oxygen or increased airflow to a patient or person in need of respiratory help.

This device consists of a lightweight tube which on one end splits into two prongs which are placed in the nostrils and from which a mixture of air and oxygen flows. The other end of the tube is connected to an oxygen supply.

Advantages:

- Gives patient oxygen
- Better for patients with claustrophobia

Disadvantages:

- Dries your nose
- Needs monitoring

During Treatment

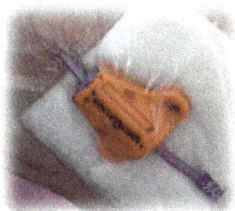

Picc line

It is a catheter that enters the body through the skin into a vein which goes to the heart through the Vena Carva. It stays in for as long as needed.

Usually used for chemotherapy and stays in whilst the patient is having it.

Advantages:

- Quick access to blood
- Easy to put IV medication down

Disadvantages:

- Cannot submerge underwater
- Constant dressing change every week

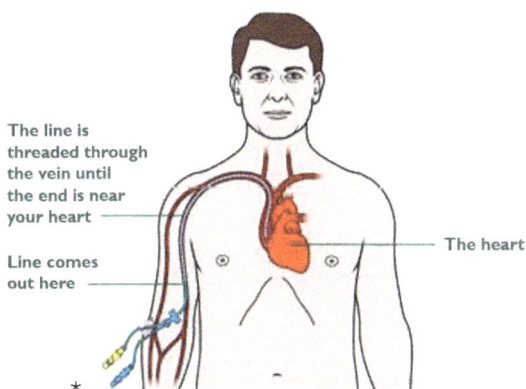

The line is threaded through the vein until the end is near your heart

The heart

Line comes out here

*

* Original illustration developed by Macmillan Cancer Support and used with permission.

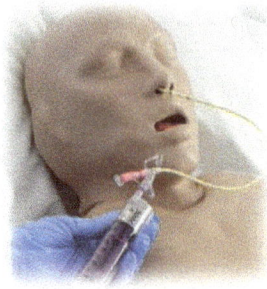

Feeding tube (NG tube)

Is an enteral feeding tube which is inserted through the nostrils down the oesophagus and into the stomach. This is usually short-term and therefore, non-invasive and not requiring surgery.

They are usually for people struggling to eat.

Advantages:

- Helps you eat when you are struggling
- Can also be used for medicine

Disadvantages:

- Can come out easily
- Not comfortable

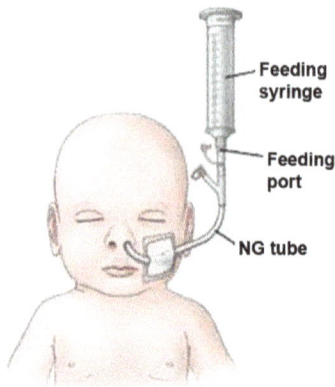

Feeding syringe

Feeding port

NG tube

Dictionary

Antibiotics
Noun
Any of a large group of chemical substances, used to treat infections.

Blood clot
Noun
A mass of coagulated/trapped blood, as within a blood vessel or at the site of an open wound.

ECHO
Medical
A machine like an ultrasound but used on your heart.

MRI
Medical
Magnetic resonance imaging; provides precise detail on a body part using magnetic fields.

CT Scan
Medical
CAT scan, provides images of the body using x-ray.

Neutrophils [*noo*-truh-fil]
Noun
White blood cell.

PET Scan
Medical
Positron emission tomography, an imaging test that uses radiotracers to assess organ and tissue functions.

Septicaemia [sep-tuh-**see**-mee-uh]
Noun pathology
Blood poisoning.

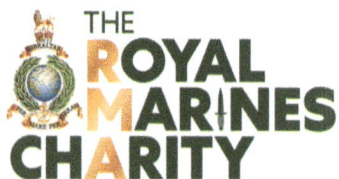
THE ROYAL MARINES CHARITY

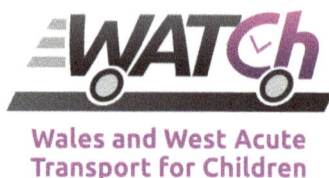
WATCh
Wales and West Acute Transport for Children

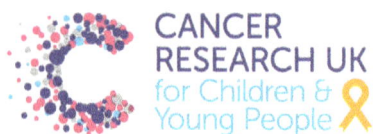
CANCER RESEARCH UK for Children & Young People

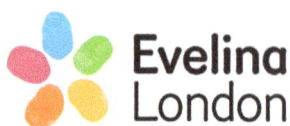
Evelina London

Thank

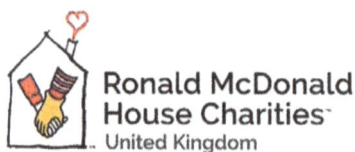
Ronald McDonald House Charities™
United Kingdom
Keeping families close™

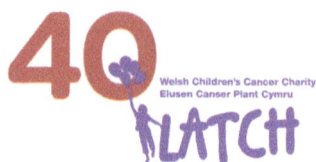
40 LATCH
Welsh Children's Cancer Charity
Elusen Canser Plant Cymru
Supporting children and their families when they need it most
Cefnogi plant a'u teuluoedd pan fydd ei angen arnynt fwyaf

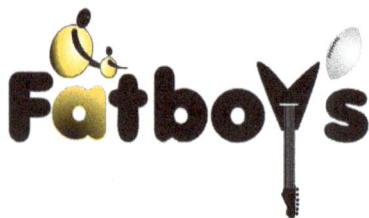
Fatboys

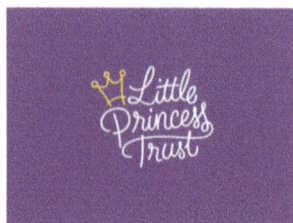
Little Princess Trust

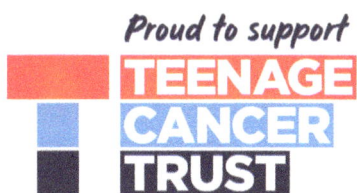

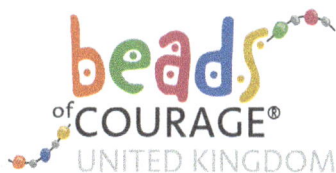

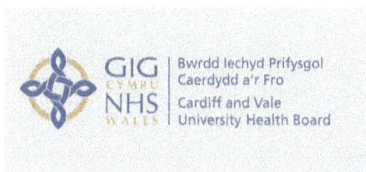

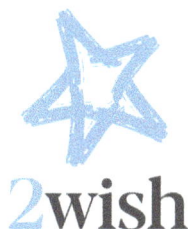

You

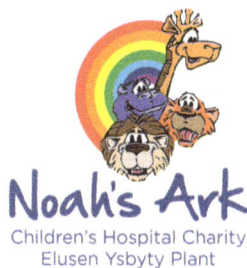

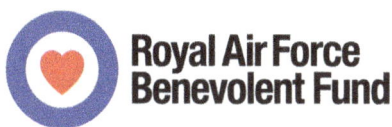

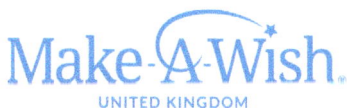

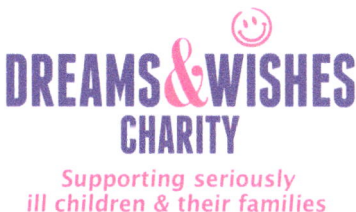

Charities

No one ever expects to go on a journey like this. A journey that changes your life in more ways than one could possibly imagine. The charities Rosie has personally thanked, made her journey and ours as a family a little more manageable.

They helped and supported us to stay together when we travelled across the UK for emergency medical care and treatment.

They took Rosie's mind off her cancer journey for a while so she could focus on healing.

They provided groundbreaking treatment and support to give her the best possible chances, and an inestimable nine months more with her we might otherwise not have had.

They helped Rosie and us create some incredible, life changing memories, when we needed them most. And they supported us when her shining light went out.

If undertaking charity fundraising this year, or you wish to donate, we ask if you could please consider one of these amazing charities.

2 Wish – Support for those affected by sudden or traumatic death in young people.
www.2wish.org.uk

Beads Of Courage UK – Spread hope, support and encouragement to seriously ill children in the UK.
https://beadsofcourageuk.org

Cancer Research UK for Children & Young People Star Awards Cancer Research UK
www.cancerresearchuk.org/children-and-young-people/star-awards

Home – Cardiff and Vale University Health Board
https://cavuhb.nhs.wales

Christie NHS Foundation Trust, Proton Beam Therapy
www.christie.nhs.uk/the-christie-charity

Dreams and Wishes Support seriously ill children and their families by creating unforgettable memories and granting lifelong wishes.
www.dreamsandwishescharity.org

Evelina London is part of Guys & St Thomas NHS foundation trust
www.evelinalondon.nhs.uk
https://evelinacharity.org.uk

Fatboys Cancer Charity for Children – Help to bring a smile to children with cancer or other life threatening illness.
www.fatboyscharity.co.uk

LATCH support children and their families who are being treated in the oncology unit a the Children's hospital for Wales.
www.latchwales.org

Make a Wish have the power to light up the darkness for children with critical illness.
www.makeawish.org.uk

Noah's Ark Children's Charity in Wales – help to ensure children and their families are cared for, with the best treatment and outcomes possible.
https://noahsarkcharity.org

Royal Air Force Benevolent Fund • Leading welfare charity – support members of the RAF family.
www.rafbf.org

Ronald McDonald House Charities – Help keep families together whilst children are in hospital.
https://rmhc.org.uk

The Royal Marines Charity – Offering lifelong support for the Royal Marines family.
https://rma-trmc.org

Teenage Cancer Trust • UK Cancer Charity – Helping young people not face cancer alone.
www.teenagecancertrust.org

Little Princess Trust – provide beautiful real hair wigs for children and young people who have lost their hair through cancer and other conditions.
www.littleprincesstrust.org.uk

The Wales and West Acute Transport for Children Service (WATCh) Bristol – provide acute management advice and inter-hospital transport for children requiring high dependency/intensive care support.
https://watch.nhs.uk

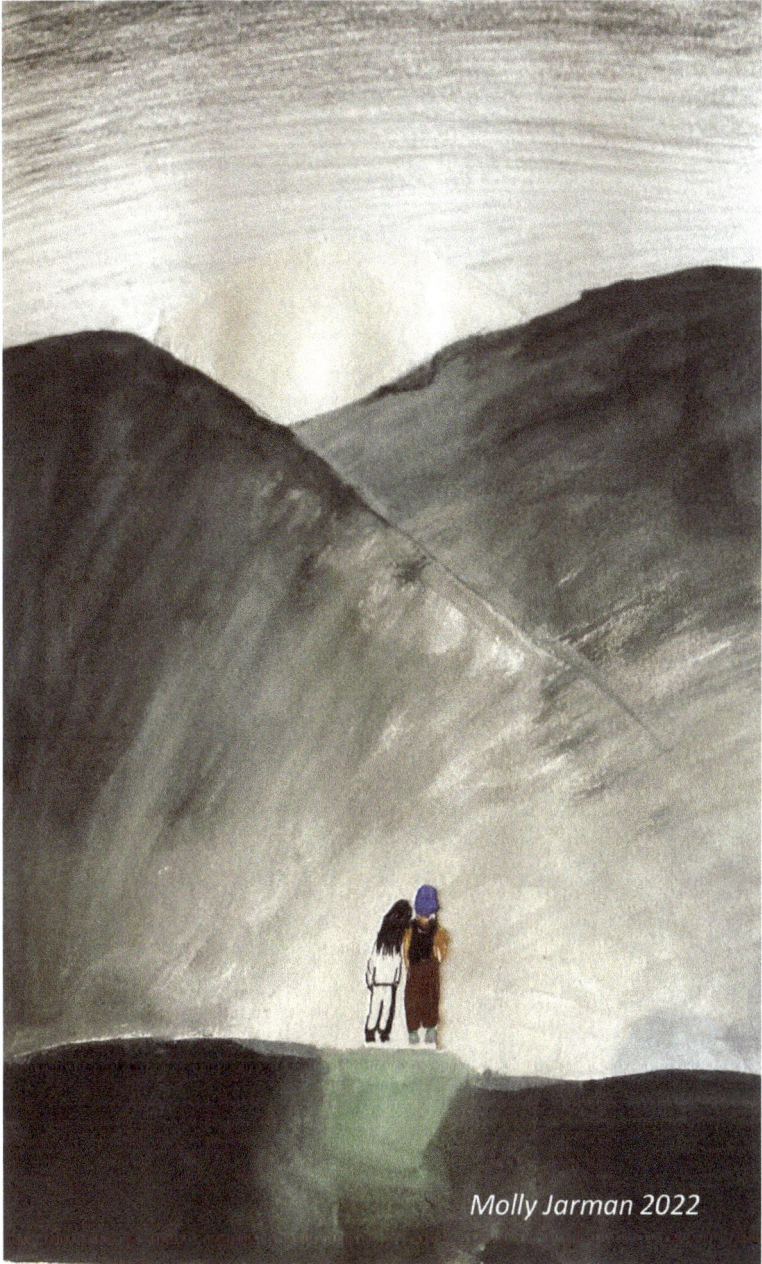

Molly Jarman 2022

References

Dear Readers, page 3

https://www.nhs.uk/conditions/cancer/

https://ukhsa.blog.gov.uk/2021/03/15/cancer-in-children-and-young-people-what-do-the-statistics-tell-us/

https://www.macmillan.org.uk/_images/carers-of-people-with-cancer_tcm9-282780.pdf

https://www.cancerresearchuk.org/health-professional/cancer-statistics-for-the-uk

Dear Diary, pages 54–61

[1] Sarcomas, Soft Tissue: Statistics | Cancer.Net
[2] Sarcoma in Children – Solving Kids' Cancer (solvingkidscancer.org)
[3] Soft Tissue Cancer — Cancer Stat Facts
[4] Hamidi M, Moody JS, Weigel TL, Kozak KR. Primary cardiac sarcoma. Ann Thorac Surg. 2010 Jul;90(1):176-81. doi: 10.1016/j.athoracsur.2010.03.065. PMID: 20609770; PMCID: PMC4201046.

Acknowledgements

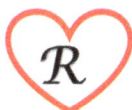

Rosie's journey was made possible thanks to all of the amazing people who work tirelessly everyday to give our children the best possible chances.

We would like to give a special mention to the following individuals including, but not exclusive to

Dr Dan the team and Dr Soha El Behery (ABUHB); Mr Conal Austin and team alongside Dr Tom, Katie and Alena (Evelina, London); Dr Madeline Adams and team alongside Julie (AMP), Gloria and Joe (Noah's Ark Children's Hospital for Wales, Cardiff and Vale UHB); Helen Clarke (LATCH); Medical team at The Christie NHS Foundation Trust Manchester, Angie (Teenage Cancer Trust) and our wonderful POONs Rachel and Nicky; Tony Curtis and team at Dreams and Wishes.

We would also like to give an extra special mention to our proton beam family who gave Rosie such joy and friendship. Sophia, Ruby and Rosie's school friends who meant everything to her.

Our family and friends who have given and continue to give us all such love and support.

Last but not least Trish Gray and her team for enabling us to share Rosie's story.

A Mountain In My Heart was written and researched in its entirety by Rosie Jarman. Supplemental 'Mummy notes' were added posthumously.

9 781789 634112